Women at Play

Women at Play

A girl's guide to everyday outdoor exercise to look good, feel good, sleep well and be happy.

Joan Griffin

Tea Trolley Press – Dublin, New Hampshire - 2010

ISBN 978-0-615-35199-5

Printed in the United States of America

www.WomenAtPlay.net

TeaTrolleyPress.com
PO Box 133
Dublin, NH 03444

This publication does not purport to give medical advice. Before
undertaking any new exercise and/or eating regimen,
consultation with your personal physician is recommended.

Cover art © Studio1340.com

Table of Contents

Introduction

Finally one thing on which we can all agree: there is one holy grail, a magic bullet, and it's exercise. New studies show no connection between reduced rates of breast cancer and a low fat diet. What does correlate with reduced rates of breast cancer? - exercise. And that's not all. A cover story in *Harvard Magazine* reported that exercise has the same effect as prescription medications used to treat depression, anxiety and sleep disorders.[1] But still many people, including women, are not physically active. Why not?

I am no amazon, much less a star athlete, but I have always been active and have never had to worry about sleeping, my weight or any of the things for which people take pills. Recently, I was at a party and a group of women were discussing diets. One turned to me and said, "You're big into running." It's true, I run regularly - 2 or 3 miles, 2 or

1. Jonathan Shaw, "The Deadliest Sin" (*Harvard Magazine*, March-April 2004, "The Power of Exercise")

3 times a week - but that's not "big into running" by anyone's standards.

It was then that I realized that I'm not big into anything. I don't race, count mileage, time myself, or measure performance (or anything else) the way people who are "big into" something usually do. I'm not big into running, I'm little into a lot of things and I do them outside and in season. Swimming, tennis and rowing in summer, skiing, ice skating and sledding in winter, hiking, biking and horseback riding in spring and fall. I participate in all of these activities at varying levels of competence, and I'm having fun; I'm not going to the Olympics anytime soon, but neither am I "taking exercise" like a dose of bad tasting medicine. I don't "work out" and I sure as heck don't do it inside at the gym.

Lately there has been a growing interest in eating a full variety of locally grown foods, in season, in reasonable portions and for pleasure. Indeed, such a lifestyle is credited for why *French Women Don't Get Fat.*[2] Food is not something to be "given up" or "taken" like a bitter pill, but something to be gathered in season and, in moderate amounts, enjoyed!

----

2. Mireille Guiliano, *French Women Don't Get Fat* (New York, Knopf, 2005).

Why shouldn't physical activity be the same? Why do you have to do one thing over and over and over again until any fun that was there has long since been drummed out of it? Why do you have to be dressed and equipped to break a world record or survive arctic conditions when there isn't much chance you're going to come anywhere near either? Why is it all so much like work? Why isn't it any fun?

I call this book *Women at Play* because the lifestyle it describes is the antithesis of the high performance competitive – or just repetitive – model, one that I think is primarily male, and I know whereof I speak. As a lawyer, I've spent my career trying civil and criminal cases, mostly against men. Winning and losing is my day job; I know Men at Work. But I also know that I've managed to stay healthy and happy while working in a profession not known for producing particularly healthy or happy people, and I very much doubt that I would have been able to do it without my regular, though moderate, outdoor exercise.

Whether in life or in exercise, my goals, like those of most women, have always been broader than just achieving the next promotion, winning the next game or logging a certain number of miles in the shortest amount of time. I want to live a natural, well-balanced life, to be as Thoreau described "well-proportioned, unstrained and standing on the soles of the feet." I don't want to be on a treadmill at work or in my personal life. While I never consciously thought I was living – or at least exercising - more like a woman than a man, lately I've begun to wonder. Maybe it's time for a new paradigm: *Women at Play*!

In this book I'll guide you through a lifestyle of seasonal outdoor activity that won't just keep you from getting fat, though it will do that, but will keep you healthy and happy, not just physically, but mentally and spiritually too. I'll show you how, by embracing a lifestyle that includes regular seasonal outdoor activity, you can overcome the real reasons so many women don't exercise even though they know that they should: they don't enjoy it and they think they don't have the time.

First, with stories of childhood summers spent in the Irish countryside in the days before TV, I'll show you just why seasonal outdoor activity is better, as well as better for you, than what is generally urged upon us as "exercise" these days – doing the same thing over and over again mostly inside at the gym or, for those without gym memberships, trudging across a grocery store parking lot or through an office stairwell. I'll show you why and how you can enjoy seasonal outdoor activities more than you ever enjoyed indoor "exercise." You'll learn that going outside is not just more fun than going to the gym, but a necessary antidote to the pressures of everyday indoor life, whether at home or on the job.

Second, I'll have a few things to say (well maybe a good few) concerning the other big reason women don't exercise – time. But unlike the so-called "authorities" on the subject, I won't urge you to "squeeze it in" while you're sitting at your desk or doing errands. Instead, I'll show you why and how, not to "make the time" – there's only so much time in the day and we can't make anymore – but to take the time for everyday outdoor exercise. You'll find, as I have, that taking the time for everyday outdoor activity is a choice that you can make. Moreover, it's a choice that you will want to make once going outside is something you enjoy and that makes you look good, feel good, sleep well and be happy.

Third, I'll give you tips and strategies for enjoying a variety of outdoor activities – focusing on those that are easy to do and easy to do close to home – by yourself or with family or friends, regardless of your and their athletic abilities. From my own experience going outside in every kind of weather, in the city, in the suburbs and out in the countryside, I'll help you decide what do to, when and where to do it, even what to wear, so exercise becomes, not something you have to do, but something you want to do.

Lastly, I will give you an easy, surefire way to help you live the lifestyle described in this book. Ask yourself, "Have I been outside today?" It's a simple question and there's only one right answer, but in that answer there's a world of variation because every season, every day is different and good for doing something outside.

So let's get started, because the sooner we do, the sooner you get to go outside and play!

1.

For Every Thing, There is a Season

Let me know what picture Nature is painting, what poetry she is writing, what ode composing now.

– H.D. Thoreau, Journals *Summer,* July 5, 1852

The best food is seasonal and so are the best outdoor activities. It's hard to argue with local strawberries available for a few brief weeks in June or a Macintosh apple picked (and eaten) in early September. Their very transience is a big part of their attraction.

Have you ever noticed how once you could record a TV show and watch it at any time, you never got around to it? You had copies of lots of shows that just weren't that compelling. Turns out part of the charm was that it was only on for a particular hour on a particular night and if you missed it you had to wait a week until it came around again. Ever wonder why you get excited to find a favorite song on the radio when you could just play it on your iPod?

Most people think it's easier to be outdoors and active if you live in Southern California or Florida where it's mild all year round, and in some ways of course they're right. But things you can do all the time can get monotonous and lose their charm. Henry Thoreau (who lived in New England) said, "Each season is incredible to the other," and wherever you have four different seasons, that's true. When I'm swimming in the lake in July, I can't imagine skating on it in January; when the lawn is buried under feet of snow in winter, I can't imagine walking barefoot over it in summer. When those things finally do roll around again, they're brand new and exciting. There is little that is year round that can compare with the smell of lilacs in the spring or the first snow right before Christmas.

Modern life, on the other hand, seems hell-bent on eradicating the seasons. I know people who keep their houses at a constant temperature winter and summer, going straight from heating to air conditioning and back again without ever opening a window. Courthouses used to be closed in August and, as recently as when I first practiced, on a hot day in July, judges on Cape Cod would let the lawyers doff their jackets to try their cases. Air conditioning has eliminated all that. T-shirts and jeans are year round attire when one stays within the confines of house, car and office.

And for some reason not entirely clear to me, as goes work, so goes play. Seasonal activities, like sailing and skiing, are replaced by treadmills, exercise bikes, rowing machines and stair masters and it's always shorts weather in the gym. Traditionally seasonal outdoor activities, like tennis and swimming, become indoor sports so they can be played all year long. My neighbor recently passed up a fine cross country ski day to go play tennis in a plastic bubble and this was not a one time event. He'll spend far more time in the bubble this winter than outside on the trails.

It strikes me that as with many things, such as food, Americans trade quality for quantity. We invented the all-you-can-eat buffet. America is a country of mediocre stuff cheap. Die-hards doggedly amass ski days and vertical feet, on man-made, machine-groomed snow, with little going for it other than predictability. I don't downhill ski many days a year by most standards, but I make a real effort to get to the mountain when it snows (how's that for radical.) A few years ago, as John and I were sitting in our respective offices on a cloudy Monday afternoon in February, John called and said it looked like our local ski hill was getting buried in snow. The next morning we did something we'd never done before, we took an unplanned day off on a Tuesday to go skiing.

When we pulled into the parking lot it was sunny and warm, which itself was unusual for a New England ski day, but we really knew this day would be different when we saw the staff digging out the lifts. There was three feet of new snow, more at the top. The lift operators were warning these New England skiers, most of whom had never seen that much powder, to stay near the one groomed path in case they had to bail out. Everyone there was playing hooky and young and old was giddy with excitement and trepidation. I wouldn't trade that day for any number of predictable ski days or vertical feet. John reminds me that I made a couple of phone calls to a client during lunch. Neither the client company nor the law firm for which I was then working survived the dot-com bust. The ski day, on the other hand, was a keeper.

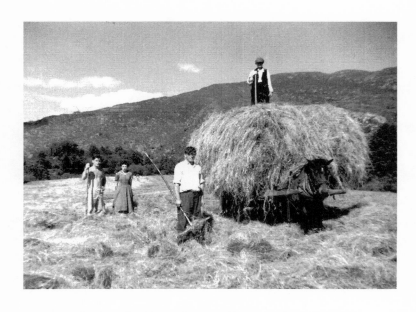

Saving the Hay, County Kerry Ireland, 1960

2.

Turnout Time

I confess that I am astonished at the power of endurance, to say nothing of the moral insensibility, of my neighbors who confine themselves to shops and offices the whole day for weeks and months, aye, and years almost together.

—   H.D. Thoreau, *Walking*

Horses are turned out every day no matter what the weather. They may also be exercised, that is ridden, but they will, in addition, be put outside in their paddocks to stand around and eat grass or hay. If horses are not turned out, they don't simply get wild or aggressive, they get anxious.

Anxiety is a modern complaint for which Americans
are taking an ever increasing and ever dehumanizing array
of drugs. Writing in the late 1800s about what was then
known as neurasthenia, Dr. George Beard described "a large
family of functional nervous disorders that are increasingly
frequent among the indoor classes of civilized countries"
particularly among "brain-working households."[3] He
considered it an essentially American disease.

My mother is from Ireland and when I was a kid we
visited my three aunts who lived with their families on three
farms in a small valley surrounded by the mountains of
County Kerry. When I first went there in the 1960s, none of
my aunts had TVs and only one had a phone. We loved to go
in June when we could help save the hay. The hay would be
cut by one of my uncles who had the tractor and cutting
machine. We would turn it by hand with pikes and leave it
to dry in the sun (hopefully). That process was repeated
several times - more times if it rained.

The hay was then made up by hand into haystacks.
When it was ready to come in, the hay was hand piked into
a wagon and brought home (originally by horse, later by
tractor) and piked up into the hay loft. I recall being a lot of

---

3. G.M. Beard, *A practical treatise on Nervous Exhaustion (Neurasthenia),*
5th ed. (New York: E.B. Treat 1905), 23, quoted in Robert D. Richardson,
William James (New York, Houghton Mifflin, 2006).

"help" standing on top and sliding down - there is no better slide than hay in the hay loft! All the while this was going on, cows had to be brought in and milked twice a day. If we went to Ireland in August rather than June, we got to go to the bog and help with the equally outdoor and labor intensive saving of the turf to burn for heat in the winter.

Needless to say after a few days of that no one was anxious. Tired and hungry, but not anxious. Not that they didn't have plenty to worry about, such as the very real possibility that it would rain and ruin everything, but the day of fresh air and physical activity prevented that legitimate worry from turning into debilitating anxiety and panic. No one had any trouble getting a good night's sleep either.

In all of the studies I have seen touting the benefits of exercise, I have never seen one that distinguishes between the indoor and outdoor varieties. Even Doctor Beard, who was observant enough in 1870 to have connected anxiety with an indoor, inactive life, missed the boat on treatment. He recommended rest, presumably indoors! Nevertheless I am convinced that there is a big difference. It's only very recently (in terms of human existence) that human beings left the farms and forests to take office jobs in the big city. The human body and mind are simply not built to sit inside all day every day typing on a computer. When my mother was growing up in Ireland, it was a treat to get into dress clothes on Sunday and sit down in church after a full week of physical outdoor work on the farm. Now most of us get dressed up everyday and sit down all the time.

Yet it's not that hard to see how we got where we are. As a child my mother really did walk the 3 (generally rainy) miles to and from school and bicycled (with no gears!) the 12 hilly miles to and from town. My uncles and cousins went up the mountain to bring the sheep down for dipping or to find a lamb who'd gone missing. When my mother and cousins left the farm, it's understandable that they gravitated toward labor saving conveniences they hadn't had growing up. And while some of my cousins have traded tending sheep for recreational hill walking, and bike riding as basic transportation for recreational cycling, many people – certainly of my parents' generation – never saw the point in going outside and tiring yourself out when you no longer had to.

The Irish experience is recent enough for me to have seen it first hand, but many American families had a similar experience back one or two generations. But in taking a well deserved rest after a hard and unpredictable life on the farm, we have collectively forgotten how, apart from the hard work, it's nice, indeed necessary, to go outside and get a little fresh air. We have thrown the baby out with the bath water.

My father is an American. He didn't grow up on a farm or have a physical job, but he has always enjoyed physical outdoor activities, work and sports. When we visited Ireland, he loved hay making! When I was growing up, every day my mother would ask my brother and me, "How was school?" When my father came home from work, however, it was a different question. Every day he wanted to know, "Did you go outside?" There was only one right answer and rather than try to defend the wrong one (a losing proposition) we - my mother, brother and I - just got into the habit of spending at least part of the afternoon outside. And more often than not my father would take us out again after dinner, playing ball or swimming in the summer, sledding or ice skating in winter, pretty exciting with Dad under the lights.

I didn't realize then that he wasn't just giving us more outdoor time; he'd had a long day inside himself and was giving himself a little turnout time too. Not too long ago I realized that subconsciously I ask myself the same question, "Have I been outside today?" Now, as then, there's only one right answer. And in case you were wondering, Dad is nothing if not consistent. Just a few weeks ago, my parents met my niece after her first day of first grade. Dad had one question, "Did you go outside for recess?" Fortunately for all concerned the answer was, "Yes!"

3.

Keep it Real

Above all, we cannot afford not to live in the present.

– H.D. Thoreau, *Walking*

Is there any real dispute that seasonal activities outside are more fun and invigorating than their indoor impostors? Can laps in an indoor chlorinated pool compare to a swim across the lake on a hot day? Does anyone really enjoy pedaling a stationary bike as much as cruising through the park or around town? How can a stationary rowing machine compare with the sheer delight (not to mention terror) of rowing in the Charles River Basin (as the duck boat blasts by)?

Outdoor activities are not just more fun than ersatz indoor ones, they are different in another obvious but significant way in that they are real. The environment is not completely controlled. You have to pay attention to where you're going and what's going on around you. You can't ride a real bike and watch TV at the same time. [Hint: If you can do it while watching TV, it's probably not worth doing.]

While you can cut yourself off from your immediate surroundings with various electronic devices, I would like to suggest you unplug. While you're paying attention to what you're doing, instead of to what some media outlet and its advertisers want you to hear or even your new favorite song, a couple of things will happen.

First, you will forget about problems at work or at home. You can't worry about the approaching duck boat or next ski bump and work at the same time and an approaching duck boat or ski bump is always a more pressing issue in the short term. This has the counterintuitive effect of allowing other problems to solve themselves and the solution to flow unbidden from your mind – for me this generally occurs around 2.5 miles into my run just as I approach the Arthur Fiedler footbridge and the final turn to home.

Second, you will notice more of the world around you, the temperature of the water or air, the feel of the wind on your face, the moon rising in the east as the sun sets in the west. You will be in the present. The natural world will take you outside of yourself and from that perspective many of your problems (even those that have not resolved themselves by the Arthur Fiedler footbridge) will seem artificial and overblown.

The London *Times* reported a recent study of high-powered people who exercised religiously at the gym under the eyes of top personal trainers, but who failed to lose weight. The study found that while these people exercised at the gym, they continued to maintain high levels of stress hormones in their bodies. Their high-powered exercise routine was as intense and stressful as their high-powered jobs - and as indoor. Is it any wonder it wasn't doing them any good? Anxiety is an indoor disease – the cure is outside.

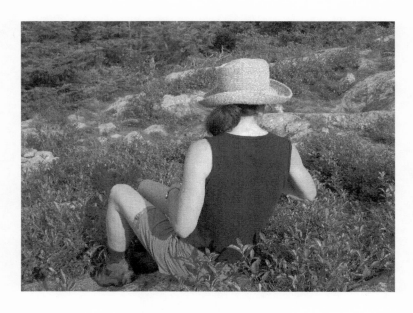

Picking wild blueberries

4.

For Every Season
There Must be a Thing
(Preferably Several)

*I believe in a different kind of division of
labor, and that Professor D. should divide
himself between the huckleberry field and
the library.*

– H.D. Thoreau, Journals *Winter*, Dec. 26, 1860

In America everyone is "big into" something – or at
least we're supposed to be. No one ever says they are
marginally into something, at least not something they've
been doing for more than a few months. If you've been
doing something for 5 or 10 years, are not particularly good
at it and aren't getting any better, maybe you should move
on to something else, right?

I've been a little into a lot of things forever, long past when I might have been expected or even encouraged to move on. I can't even say I used to be great (like in college) but my game has gotten rusty due to obligations of work and family. In fact, I was never a particularly gifted athlete and I'm pretty much as good as I've ever been (or am likely to get) at most things. I have not been and am not now going to the Olympics. (And let me say for the record, I would have loved to have gone – walking in the opening ceremonies, standing humbly on the dais while the flag was raised and the anthem played . . .)

Although you will not find me in the record books, there are benefits to moderation. I have no repetitive stress injuries, not having repeated any one activity all that much! Even running, my mainstay physical outdoor activity in all seasons, I only do 2 or 3 times a week, 2 or 3 (flat) miles a day. I did enough running in high school to know that 9 miles a week doesn't qualify anyone for a subscription to *Runner's World*, but I also knew that the physical and mental benefits of 9 miles a week far outweighed 0 miles, so that is what I have done, quietly and for years. Recently a friend who has worked as a personal trainer said, "Three threes - that's all you need to get all of the major benefits of running." Who knew!

Let's face it, doing one thing over and over again sounds like work, repetitive factory-type work at that. Indeed, at the dawn of the industrial revolution, a school of philosophers argued that lack of variety at work was bad for human beings, tuning them into little more than machines as compared with the well-rounded farmers and small businessmen of previous generations. Thoreau urged the professor to "divide his time between the huckleberry field and the library," still good advice today if you can figure out how to make a living at the same time. But even if specialization is a fact of life at work, why self impose it on our play?

When I graduated from high school and was applying to college, the ideal student was well-rounded, with classes and activities spanning a variety of academic subjects, sports, art or music and leadership positions. Now it seems the opposite is true. Parents push their children to excel at one sport or musical instrument. If the child can't be a star in more popular sports, ambitious parents urge him or her to choose little known ones so there be less competition and the child will stand out. Even very talented athletes who a generation ago would have played football or soccer, basketball and baseball each in its season, must specialize in one and play it all year round before they are even out of grade school.

The loss of the well-rounded person living a well-rounded life is a shame. The failure to prepare our kids to live a balanced life is inexcusable. None of these kids, except a very few, is going to the Olympics. Many more, unfortunately, will develop repetitive stress injuries before they are even out of high school which will put an end to their competitive careers and, what is far worse, limit their ability to enjoy physical activity throughout their lives. Those who cannot compete at the semi-professional level that is scholastic sports are discouraged from any physical activity and relegated to video games.

I actually think a lot of kids would agree. I've often noticed that kids who played competitive sports all their young lives really seem to enjoy intramural sports in college. They seem relieved when they can no longer make the varsity team. They don't miss the grueling practices or spending all weekend traveling to tournaments which their mothers apparently enjoyed more than they did. They enjoy the physical activity and the friendly competition of a weekly game as part of a balanced life, not as the whole of an unbalanced one.

I have nothing against competition, just the amount of time it takes to be competitive these days. For a (short) while I competed in horse shows with the horse I rode a few times a week. I know of no sport where the time spent packing up for and getting to the event so far exceeds the time spent actually competing. Then when you're done, you can't just go get a drink or watch the other competitors, you have to take care of the horse! (Not to mention pack him up and take him home.) After a couple of such marathon Sundays, John offered me a deal I couldn't refuse. He'd build me a few fences in the yard and once a week I could ride around the course and he'd give me a blue ribbon!

Once we accept that we are not going to the Olympics (and maybe not even the club or town championship), our options multiply dramatically. If you live in an area that has all four seasons, and if you embrace a lifestyle of seasonal activities outdoors, you will by definition participate in a variety of them, since you can't go skiing in the summer or swimming in the winter. If you live where it's warm all the time and you can do the same things all year round, make your own seasons and change out activities accordingly. Do as the ladies in Puerto Rico do at Christmastime and wear your velvet, even if it is 70 balmy degrees (but maybe forgo the mink!)

5.

Exercise is Not Medicine;
Life is Not a Disease

*But the walking of which I speak has nothing
in it akin to taking exercise, as it is called, as
the sick take medicine at stated hours, – as the
swinging of dumbbells or chairs; but is itself
the enterprise and adventure of the day.*

– H.D. Thoreau, *Walking*

I recently saw an interview of a prestigious doctor who specializes in recovery, not only from cancer, but from cancer treatment. As it was late December she was asked what she would recommend to people for the coming year. She said if she could recommend only three things she would recommend a balanced diet, sleep and exercise. So far so good. But then she got specific. She advised each person to buy a pedometer and walk 10,000 steps a day.

Nothing against walking (I love a nice walk) but recommendations like that are why I am writing this book. My other favorite recommendations from so-called health experts are parking your car at the far end of the grocery store parking lot or climbing stairs at the office. Who wants to spend their precious free time in a parking lot or stair well? No one, which is why nobody does it.

Exercising our bodies should not be as joyless as taking the car in for an oil change. Actually, even car maintenance is a lot more fun that that doctor's recommendation. I have an old convertible that gets an annual check up in the spring. I wasn't really sure what was involved so I called up to see how it was going. It was one of the first sunny warm days of the spring and after they had changed the oil, they had taken the car out (top down of course) for a fast drive to "clean out" the engine. I have since learned that this is known in the trade as an "Italian tune-up." Now that sounds like fun! If it sounds fun to you throw out the pedometer and take yourself out (top down!) for an Italian tune-up too.

Variety is the key to keeping things fun. Whether it's returning to an old favorite at the start of a new season or taking up something entirely new, the novelty is part of the enjoyment. If you do decide to take up something new, although it may take some initial effort, remember to have fun while you're at it. When beginners are learning to ride a horse, they're always allowed to canter early on so they have some fun and feel that making the effort to learn will be worthwhile.

Once I had to step in and teach the last day of an adult swimming class at the YWCA. Everyone in the class had passed the Beginners' test so they all could swim the length of the pool. I suggested they use their new hard won skills (learning to swim as an adult is very worthwhile but not easy) to have a little fun and jump off the diving board. One young woman wasn't confident that someone as small as I could save her if need be. So she insisted I gather up *all* the safety equipment – life ring, shepherd's crook and anything else that was around - before she jumped. She had me so overburdened that I was more likely to drown myself than be of any use to her, but it gave her the confidence she needed to jump off the board and I already knew she could swim herself to the side. She did – they all did – and they had a blast. I really think that until that moment they had forgotten why they had wanted (and had worked so hard) to learn to swim.

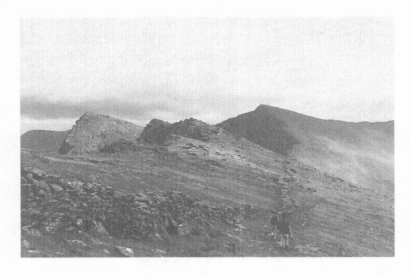

Mt. Brandon, Dingle, Ireland

6.

Looking Good

But greatness is well-proportioned,
unstrained and stands on the soles of the feet.

   −   H.D. Thoreau, Journals *Early*
         Spring, Feb. 26, 1840

Different people enjoy different kinds of activities for a variety of different reasons. I choose my activities for reasons seldom urged in either the performance-oriented single sport magazines or the fear-mongering medical journals. For example, I'm always attracted to things that have the potential to make me look good - both while I'm doing it and after. Anyone who has ever taken a walk on a brisk day knows what the activity and the exposure does for the complexion. Some years ago I realized that I looked best − younger, healthier, prettier − when I looked in the mirror of the very rustic bathroom at the barn just after riding my horse. The place I look worst? Hands down in the fluorescent light of the law office! Looking at myself in the ladies' room mirror, my skin is pasty, my eyes are dull, I look like I'm going to die! (Note to self, ride more, work less, at least in the office!) But again, while we may be stuck (at least in the short term) with work and the work environment, what we do on our own time is up to us.

I like to do things that make me look elegant, in balance and taller! But that doesn't limit me to ballet dancing or yoga (although I suspect that looking good is a major part of yoga's appeal for many women). John has a nephew who was a star basketball and football player in high school. At his parents' house hanging on the wall there is a picture of him preparing to shoot a basketball. He is relaxed, his weight is slightly back on his heels, his eyes are on the hoop. You can draw a straight line from his shoulder, through his hip and to his heel, the perfect posture of equestrians and ballet dancers. Patrick, who also played college football for Notre Dame, is not much of a ballet dancer, but in this picture he is tall, elegant, and in balance. He looks good (and I'll bet he made that shot).

Looking good naturally brings up the question of attire, a subject that will be addressed in greater detail later, but in general, let me begin by saying that you don't have to invest in lots of single sport gear to play outside year round.

On the contrary, my apologies to the sportswear industry, you can wear a lot of the same clothes doing a variety of activities. No one is going to send you home because you're out of uniform and since we're not playing at a semi-professional level or in extreme conditions, we don't need that much specialized equipment or clothing.

My personal yardstick is if you can't see Audrey Hepburn wearing it, it's probably not a good idea. Men like to look like they've just emerged from a war zone – the more gear, gadgets and pockets the better. This is not a good look for most women, especially petite women like me. Only the tall (and preferably buxom) can get away with bulging exterior pockets below the waistline. Most of us simply can't carry all that "extreme." We don't look taller, stronger, sleeker. We look like we're about to go down for the third time. And if you look that way, chances are you feel that way, and are neither doing very well nor having much fun, and the odds are you won't be back anytime soon (and why should you be, you look crummy!)

But, you might ask, if I don't wear regulation attire no one will take me seriously? Well, I answer, that is exactly the point. You are out there to get some exercise, fresh air and have fun. You don't take yourself seriously so you sure as heck don't want anyone else doing it (mainly because then you might get confused and take yourself seriously too.)

As a rule of thumb, if you look like the pride of a nation (or at least a major metropolitan region) is riding on your next move, you're wearing too much regulation attire.

My mother tells of being out for a drive one day in the 1940s with her father's American cousin (a priest) who was visiting Ireland. As she proudly pointed out the local 3000 foot mountain, perhaps suggesting greater familiarity with the climb up than was strictly warranted, he pulled over to the side of the road and said, "Race you to the top!" Off they went in whatever they were wearing at the time, he in his priest's collar and she in her skirt and sensible shoes.

Here in New Hampshire, Mount Monadnock is said to be one of the most frequently climbed mountains in the world because it's the closest one to Boston. On a nice summer weekend, most kids head up in T-shirts and sneakers, but there are always a few people decked out in full high tech regalia. I wonder what they'd think if they saw the pictures of the turn of the century ladies in their long skirts, white high neck blouses and lace up boots enjoying the view from the top (and looking, by the way, very good)?

7.

It's Not a Numbers Game

There is something servile in the habit of seeking after a law which we may obey. We may study the laws of matter at and for our convenience, but a successful life knows no law.

– H.D. Thoreau, *Walking.*

Recently a neighbor sent me a book by a famous and well-respected doctor. In it, the famous doctor explained a detailed and regimented exercise program which sought to imitate natural activity like running after the dog up and down hills. I offer no regimented program. I simply do natural activities, like running up and down hills!

Everyone wants a magic bullet, a pill, a set of rules that will fix everything – "a law which we may obey." But we are not 19th century yokels willing to believe the claims of just any "patent medicine" or elixir. We want our cure to be reliable. We want it to be backed by a scientific study that tells us not just what to do, but the proven mechanism of how and why it's going to work.

The only problem is, historically at least, pretty much all of the scientifically proven truths based on studies have turned out to be wrong. Remember when we weren't supposed to eat butter because margarine was better for us? Remember when cholesterol was bad before they found out that at least some of it is actually good? And none of this was all that long ago.

I am all for science. I have an undergraduate degree in engineering. Litigating patent cases I have worked my way through a lot of scientific problems. But maybe because of that, more than most people, I am willing to look under the covers of so-called scientific studies and look critically at what is being proffered as established fact.

It's not really surprising that these studies were wrong or that over time we learn more that helps us understand things differently. That is to be expected. What amazes me is that no sooner do we learn that the last study was wrong, than we are prepared to take the next study as gospel truth. And in my experience no one is more gullible when it comes to scientific studies than doctors. I have some very smart friends doing medical research at the very best hospitals in this country and yet they seem more vulnerable to unquestioning belief in the latest scientific study than the least educated among us.

One such friend was visiting with his family and as I put salt on the table he said that the kids couldn't eat salt because it was bad for them. I'm sure I rolled my eyes or did something equally disrespectful and his wife (the doctor) said, "It's okay, I've read a new study." He said, "Why didn't you tell me!" While I was delighted for the kids that they could eat moderate amounts of salt, I couldn't help wonder why, if the old study was wrong, she was so confident that the new one was right.

The problem as I see it with all of these studies is that they are typically very narrow, studying just one factor and its effect on one aspect of the human body. They almost never consider, and perhaps wouldn't be able to consider, all of the other factors that interact with whatever is being studied and its ultimate effect, not just on one measurement, like fat or cholesterol, but on the whole person.

I think it's safe to say that we may never fully understand how the human body and mind, heart and soul all work together. But what we must not do is base our behavior on the results of piecemeal studies (often paid for by somebody selling something – like margarine!)

I do what works and makes sense for me even though I may not fully understand how or why it works. I always ate butter and just knew there had to be something wrong with all of that fake stuff. I never believed that one cholesterol number determined whether I was healthy or not. I was never tempted by the supposed convenience of the office tower matrix of work, cafeteria and indoor gym.

Nor do I need or even want to convert my life into a series of technical requirements. I have never measured how fast I run or ride, much less my heart rate at mile 2 or 10. I sometimes get the feeling that the more that's measured, the less that's actually getting done. Ask anyone who's worked out on a stair machine or treadmill and they will tell you those 10 stories or 5 miles they supposedly climbed or ran are nothing compared with the real thing. Run or bike to the top of a hill to get a view and you won't need to measure anything to know you've gotten a workout. If you need to talk about cardio and carbs to show that you're serious about your health, go ahead. But, as for me, a morning hike and waffles with maple syrup will do just fine.

I know from my own experience that regular exercise and time outside are necessary in order to keep me healthy and happy, and they have kept me that way despite working in a profession not well known for producing particularly healthy or happy people. I believe the studies –

as long as the results are consistent with my experience, otherwise I maintain a healthy skepticism.

I recently ran into the neighbor who had given me that complicated program mimicking natural activities. He said he gave it up after about two weeks. Last I heard he was back out on the trails running up and down the hills!

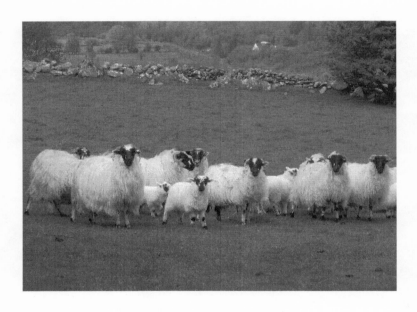

Lambs in the field, Ireland

8.

Men Playing with
Women at Play

Like overtasked school boys, all my members
and nerves and sinews petition thought for a
recess, and my very thigh bones itch to slip
away from under me, and run and join in the
melee.

— H.D. Thoreau, Journals *Winter,*
Jan. 24, 1841

You might think that to engage in a variety of
outdoor activities at a moderate and uncompetitive level
would require other, presumably female, companions with
the same goals as yourself. Yes, but not necessarily.

Men, and indeed anyone who fancies him or herself
a competitive athlete, are only too delighted to have you as
an excuse to take the whole thing down a notch. So for

example after a moderate morning hike where you don't get to the top of anything or an invigorating 15 mile bike ride that is far short of a "century," your husband, boyfriend, competitive male or female friend can honestly tell his or her other competitive friends that they would have loved to have gone farther, faster or longer but couldn't because you were along.

What a nice break for them. When my 6' 2", 180 pound husband does the same activity as I do some morning or afternoon, I will be going pretty much to the limit of my ability while he is barely exerting any effort at all!

Even better, you can turn what looks like a liability into an asset. If you are hiking, biking, canoeing or doing just about anything with someone who is bigger and stronger than you are, and more to the point wants to prove it by doing something more strenuous, let him! He can carry more on a hike, ride in front of you into the wind on a bike ride or do much more than his fair share of paddling a canoe. I myself have gone farther, faster and longer than I ever would have on my own because John was doing the lion's share of the work.

Again, the advantages go both ways. If you've ever read in the newspapers about weekend hikers lost in the mountains in a snow storm having gone farther and stayed out later than was sensible, you will almost always find that the participants were men. If a woman had been along, she would have very sensibly refused to go so far or so long and insisted they turn for home at a reasonable hour. Most importantly, the guy she was with could then have headed home himself at a reasonable hour because it was her idea.

In fact, since most families and groups of friends are comprised of members of different sizes and strengths, ages and abilities, it's always useful to be able to accommodate a variety of skill sets in as many activities as possible. The standard response may be for everyone to go his or her separate way, Mom to yoga, Dad to the gym, brother and sister to their respective class or team sport. But wouldn't it be nice (not to mention less time consuming) if we could all play together? To that end, for most activities discussed below, I suggest specific strategies that have worked for John and me to bridge the (considerable) gap between us to allow us to play together.

9.

If it's Not for You, Don't do it

A man does best when he is most himself.

– H.D. Thoreau, Journals *Winter*, Jan. 21, 1852

Variety is great, but just as with food, there will be some things that are just not for you. If, after giving something a reasonable try, you really don't enjoy it, move on to something else. It's called play for a reason!

There are a number of perfectly good activities that just don't appeal to me, so I don't do them (but of course, you may!) Kayaking, for example, too plastic, too low, too confined, give me a canoe any day. Ditto roller blading. Anything that requires donning that much padding clearly involves too much unwelcome contact with hard surfaces to be attractive to me and as for looking good, let's just say no politician or sitting judge should allow him or herself to be photographed in roller blading gear. Also roller blading just feels slow to me. I'd rather ride a bike.

Golf is also probably not my thing. John plays but has discouraged me from taking it up. My favorite part of tennis is running after the ball and there's not a lot of that in golf. Actually most of the things I enjoy involve movement and in golf there's a lot of standing still, very very still.

So if you find yourself not having much fun, don't suffer in silence, get out of there. Last spring my friend Valerie, a fellow defense attorney and avid tennis player, joined her husband, an avid golfer, on a vacation to Scarsdale, Arizona. Valerie's intent was to take up golf as it was such a focus of her husband's free time, and given that she is active and reasonably well coordinated, she didn't anticipate a problem. But halfway through day two, as she and her husband and two other couples were out on the course heading into the back nine, she decided golf was not for her. So when she spied a passing maintenance cart, to hear her husband tell it, she stood up and waved her arm "like she was flagging a cab in New York City." As she climbed into the cart she asked the surprised groundskeeper, "Are you going back to the clubhouse? I'm done here."

10.

Take the Time

*A broad margin of leisure is as beautiful in a
man's life as in a book.*

 −   H.D. Thoreau, Journals *Winter,* Dec. 28, 1852

I recently saw one of my Irish cousins who'd grown
up working hard on his family's farm but now like most Irish
has a desk job in Dublin. I asked him whether his son (then
17) would have a job for the summer. He said, "Oh he would
love to, but he hasn't the time." Apparently his summer was
already booked with scouting trips to France, orienteering in
Scotland and a vacation in China with his mother! I aspire to
be him. Someday I too will say, "I would love to have a job,
but I haven't the time." Until then, however, I, like most
people, must fit in my outside time around office work,
cooking, cleaning, grocery shopping, bill paying (OK John

actually does the bills, but you get the idea) and everything else it takes to keep life going. So now you know that outdoor exercise is a good idea, but how to fit it in?

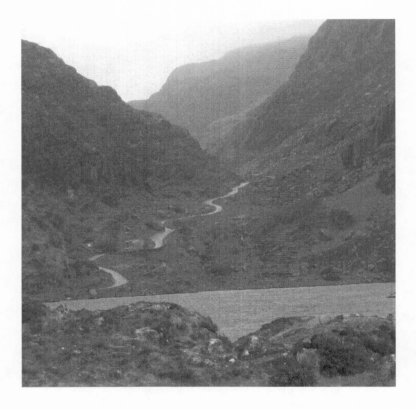

Gap of Dunloe, County Kerry, Ireland

A.

You can't "Squeeze" it in

*In my afternoon walk I would fain forget all
my morning occupations and my obligations
to society. But it sometimes happens that I
cannot easily shake off the village. The
thought of some work will run in my head
and I am not where my body is, – I am out of
my senses. In my walks I would fain return to
my senses.*

> – H.D. Thoreau, *Walking*

Daily it seems we are bombarded with suggestions to "squeeze" in exercise while we're working, talking on the phone or (heaven forbid!) driving the car. I know of a furniture company that is designing office furniture so you can exercise at your desk. Another recent article touted the benefits of typing on your laptop as you run on the treadmill, though they did say you had to be careful not to let the treadmill get away from you as you focus on your screen. Boy does that sound like fun.

I will simply say that in my experience that kind of multitasking (actually most multitasking) doesn't work. Indeed, I would guess it just makes things worse. Why? You're still at your desk worried and under stress from whatever it is you're working on and now you've just added the pressure of one more totally incompatible thing. If, as those personal trainers found in London, stress hormones just keep pumping when your exercise is as high stress as your work, imagine the hormones when you exercise while you work! Whatever the actual mechanism, that approach - trying to squeeze in yet another activity into an already overcrowded life - isn't going to work. You can't multitask your way to health and well-being. The whole point of outdoor exercise is to get the mind as well as the body away from all of life's indoor "tasks" and the stress they all too often generate.

So if I am not suggesting squeezing outdoor exercise into an already overcrowded life, what am I suggesting? I'm suggesting making regular outdoor activity part of a balanced healthy lifestyle. What that requires will vary from person to person. For some, it will be a simple reordering of priorities; for others it may require more structural changes that can't be completely accomplished overnight. But for everyone, the process can be begun. If weekday outdoor activity is impractical due to long work hours or commutes, at the very least one half day each weekend can be set aside for vigorous outdoor fun. Once the benefits are apparent, the ability to enjoy regular outdoor activity, like access to good schools or proximity to good medical care, will start to inform all of life's decisions, including where to live and where to work.

For most people, regular outdoor exercise is within reach. If you can't easily fit it into your day, keep a diary of how you spend your time, just as you might keep a diary of the food you eat or money you spend if you were trying to get a handle on diet or budget. It's likely this exercise will reveal "empty calories," things that take time but contribute little to your or your family's well being. Too frequent trips to Target or unplanned trips to the grocery store come to mind. A trip to the store to pick up a single item takes at least a half an hour which you could have spent outside. Make weekly shopping trips, and if you've forgotten an ingredient, substitute something you do have – it will probably turn out fine and maybe you'll even come up with something new!

Your diary may also reveal "budget busters," such as limitless hours driving other people (presumably your children) to what they want to do at the expense of your having any time to do what you want and in fact need to do for yourself. I have never understood why American children are presumed to be entitled (in fact required) to participate in no end of athletic and other activities while adults (namely their parents) are relegated to working and car pooling to support their fantasy lifestyle. What is the point of those children becoming so highly trained in extracurricular activities if all it leads to is a life of working long hours and carpooling? Perhaps our kids would be better served if they saw in the adults around them a good example of living a balanced life.

The truth is everyone would benefit from a better balance. Some years ago there was an article in our local paper about a family that noticed they no longer went hiking together as they had when the kids were younger because they were spending all of their afternoons and weekends at soccer. They made the radical decision to take their kids out of soccer so they could all spend more time together as a family doing a greater variety of outdoor activities.

This is a difficult decision to make if the child likes soccer and everyone else is doing it. But the point is to understand that you are making a choice, and not simply go along with a program that may not be right for you or your family. Even if soccer or dance or some other time-consuming activity isn't eliminated entirely, a family can decide that the child will play on the local school team but not the club team that travels and practices all year long and recapture that time for other activities.

Although things may seem more complicated now, and in some ways they are, the truth is there has always been a lot to do and choices to be made among many options. I had a friend growing up who was a good athlete. At a time when Title IX was just beginning to make sports available to girls, she excelled at gymnastics, tennis, skiing and softball. While we were in high school she had the opportunity to go to a full-time, live-in gymnastics training camp run by a famous Olympic coach. My friend's father counseled her against the extreme dedication to one sport. Although she was good for our school, it's unlikely she would have made it to the Olympics or even to a career in college. He urged her to play at the high school level and to play all of the sports she enjoyed – in other words to be a balanced athlete and person.

When I went to college I met another girl who had attended that full-time gymnastics program. As a result of an injury, her career was over and she didn't even compete at the college level. I was surprised at the time that she didn't seem to mind leaving it all behind. I have since decided that my friend's father was a wise man.

B.

Just because you can, doesn't mean you should

Nothing can be more useful to a man than a determination not to be hurried.

— H.D. Thoreau, Journals *Early Spring*, Mar. 22, 1842

There isn't much to which this doesn't apply, from all-you-can-eat buffets to all night e-mail access. While some candidates for overindulgence, such as the former, may be obvious and therefore more easily avoided, others, such as the latter, are more insidious and creep up on you unexpectedly.

As modern life creates more opportunities to do more things more often it's up to us to regulate ourselves. We can no longer rely on the blue laws to keep us from spending our Sundays in the shopping mall. We can no longer rely on locked office buildings to keep us from working seven days a week. We can no longer rely on rainy days to keep us from overindulging in what were once outdoor sports like tennis and swimming.

A recent article noted that horse shows had so proliferated in the last 20 years that a horse could now be shown every weekend, while in former years he could only have been shown once a month. The author noted, "Everything has changed, except the horse."[4] What he meant was that the horse's body could not withstand the excessive show schedule and heavy practice that went with it. But many horse owners and riders simply assumed that if a show were on, they should go. A clear case of "just because you can, doesn't mean you should."

What's true for horses is equally true for people. While everything else may have changed, we haven't changed much at all. We still need eight hours of sleep a night, three meals a day and regular outdoor exercise. The world may operate on a 24/7 schedule, but no one of us can for any period of time.

Except in the cases of professional athletes, our bodies are not built to withstand the amount of repetitious activity now permitted by constant availability. (Indeed what separates professional athletes from the rest of us is not

4. Jim Wofford, *Practical Horseman*, 2009.

just their skill at their sport but the fact that their bodies can withstand the amount of practice it takes to get to that level.) Most of us are not built to swing a tennis racket for hours on end all year round. Our knees don't benefit from the amount of downhill skiing you can now do in a day in the age of high-speed lifts. It's up to us to decide, not whether we can, but whether we should.

This applies to, and affects, every area of our lives. Even things that seem fun and convenient can turn out to be too much of a good thing. Low-cost airfares make it possible to travel great distances for short periods of time – for a weekend, to attend a graduation – trips that would not have been possible just a generation ago. But these conveniences come at a cost. Lots of time in airplanes and the inevitable delay in airports doesn't constitute a relaxing or restorative weekend or vacation. And a flying visit for a weekend is no substitute for those three week vacations we used to take back when flying to Ireland was a big deal. Sometimes it will be worth it, but other times it won't be. The problem is, if you assume you should, simply because you can, you will be stuck with both.

Anyone who wishes that there were more hours in the day is trying to do too much and probably not enjoying any of it. We must take it as a given, like the options in the all-you-can-eat buffet, that there are more things you might like to do in a day than you can reasonably fit in. Armed with that knowledge, we can make better choices.

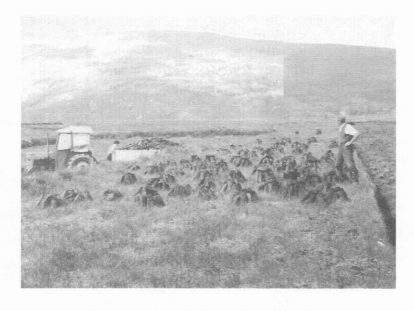

Footing the turf, County Kerry, Ireland

C.

Just because everyone else does, doesn't mean you have to

Be so little distracted, your thoughts so little confused, your attention so free, your existence so mundane, that in all places and in all hours you can hear the sound of crickets in seasons when they are to be heard.

— H.D. Thoreau, Journals *Summer, July 7, 1851*

If some aspect of your life is crowding out the basic necessities, balanced diet, sleep and outdoor exercise, the first step is admitting there is a problem. The next is deciding what to do about it. The vast majority of people who live unbalanced lives simply take as a given long days at the office, long commutes and equally out-of-control children's schedules.

Even things that seem to be required are for the most part optional. The important thing is to realize that we are always making choices. You don't want to get to the end of your life and find out you've been having someone else's version of a good time!

I recently saw an article discussing the results of a survey on how Americans spend their time. Not surprisingly most Americans claim they are short of time. The survey showed that Americans spend less time with their spouses, less time eating as a family and less time with their families as a whole. But there is one category where there is plenty of time, indeed an increase rather than decrease in time spent. That category is watching television. The average American spends two to three hours a day watching TV (and that probably doesn't even count surfing the internet or playing video games), plenty of time to go outside and have some fun.

We don't have a TV and haven't had one for over 10 years. Obviously, in this day and age that would seem to be an extreme decision and, of anything I've ever done, going "TV less" is the one that draws the most comment from anyone who hears it. I think it didn't seem such a foreign idea to me because I had been to farms in Ireland that had no TVs, and it didn't seem to me then, and it doesn't seem to me now, that we suffered without them. I remember conversation, music, visits, soccer games in an empty (hopefully) field on the long summer nights, nothing I would trade for a night in front of the television. So I was not surprised by another recent study reporting that watching more TV doesn't make anyone any happier.[5]

John says he gives people credit who watch TV, he doesn't know how they find the time! Although women watch plenty of TV, my guess is they are less attached to it than are the men in their lives. When I have told women friends that we don't have a TV, more than one has responded that she would gladly give it up to get her husband out from in front of theirs! I think one reason people watch so much TV, more than they realize, is that they are tired and drained from the rest of their day and can't muster the energy to do anything else.

Although it's counterintuitive, daily outdoor exercise increases, rather than decreases, energy. The increase in energy from taking a break from work and spending some time doing physical activity outdoors makes tasks that might otherwise seem difficult or daunting easier. The result is you get more done in less time. I often think that my daily and weekly outdoor activity saves time in the end and I know it improves the quality of my work.

Excessive TV watching is also symptomatic of a larger problem. We have become a nation of spectators rather than doers. TV, movies, sports, music, there is so

---

5. Jonathan Clements, "Getting Going", *The Wall Street Journal*, April 2, 2008.

much opportunity to watch or listen to star performances by someone else that we have pretty much given up doing much of anything (except our jobs) ourselves. Not so many years ago if you wanted music after dinner, someone in the family had to play it on the piano and everyone else was expected to sing. If you wanted to show someone a nice view you'd seen on vacation, you had to draw a picture of it "en plein air." Plays and ball games were things you did as least as much as watched. And when you did watch, it was your friends and neighbors in person not international stars continents away whom you will never meet (and who will never watch you!)

I remember much more doing than spectating when we visited Ireland in the 1960s. Out in the country, with no TVs and not much recorded music in the house, everyone did something - played the accordion or tin whistle, sang, danced, recited poetry or told stories - and was called upon to give his or her "party piece" as the entertainment for the evening. In the days before electronics, there was a lot of singing while you worked in the fields and around the farm. While some people were more talented than others (and were invited to more parties!) participation in sports or music was not limited to up and coming stars, as it would be today. It was just a part of everyday life.

Now with essentially limitless opportunities to watch and listen to really amazing performances there is seemingly no time, and even less inclination, to learn, practice and participate ourselves. But watching someone else do something, however well, is a poor substitute for doing something yourself, however poorly. It may seem presumptuous to skip a televised match of the top tennis players in the world in favor of batting the ball around the local courts yourself, but unless you have unlimited time that may well be a choice you should make and at least you'll know the courts will be free!

Unfortunately, for many people, watching TV, eating out and shopping are the only "recreation" they know. New housing developments, particularly in the south and west, have big houses with huge indoor playrooms for the kids and media rooms – and indoor theaters! – for the whole family. Indoor playrooms are filled with equipment – like playhouses and slides – that when I was growing up was only to be found outside. And despite bucolic sounding names like "The Estates at Green Acres," there is no place within walking distance for daily outdoor exercise much less contact with nature.

The fact that people nowadays will buy big-box houses with no access to the outdoors shows just how out of balance our lives have become. What was once a common everyday occurrence is now a completely foreign idea.

There is a lot that was once common sense that seems to have gotten lost in modern life and, conversely, much that is generally accepted now that doesn't make much sense. A few years ago when we were on our annual family ski trip, my brother had the TV on in the ski condo. Being TV less at home, I hadn't seen it in a while. Good Morning America was on and Katie Couric was interviewing a young woman about a new diet program. The young woman wore a white lab coat and held a plastic tray divided into three sections. She had different types of food in each section of the tray. She explained to Katie quite seriously that the really remarkable thing about this new diet was that you could combine foods from different parts of the tray into a single meal.

Then she gave an example. She said you could take one of your carbohydrates, at this she picked up a slice of bread, add to it your protein, at this she picked up a slice of turkey, and then take yet another carbohydrate, here she picked up another slice of bread, and combine these different food groups to form a single meal. The woman had created a turkey sandwich. I was dumbfounded that this was being shown in all seriousness on TV as a "new and revolutionary diet," but there was Katie Couric nodding solemnly as it was explained to her. From the kitchen as he was preparing our lunches John chimed in, "Well now I know why my sandwiches weren't working. I've only been using one carbohydrate!"

When a turkey sandwich is being presented as revolutionary by a woman in a white lab coat, you know we've taken a wrong turn somewhere and it was a good ways back. Much that is considered normal now is completely wrongheaded and downright foolish. There is a lot of nonsense out there and one goes along with it unquestioningly at one's peril. Happily the best plan is usually the simple, obvious one that requires no white lab coat or complicated program. What it does take is a willingness to recognize that how you live is a matter of choice and a willingness to make your choices consciously, however unconventional by today's standards they may be.

So ask yourself, "How much TV do you really want to watch? How much time do you want to spend shopping? How much time do you want to spend spectating rather than doing?" Try substituting regular outdoor activity for any of these and I doubt you will say that your time would have been better spent in front of the television, on the computer or at the mall.

D.

*You're not the f*ing red cross!*

Staying in the house breeds a sort of insanity always.

– H.D. Thoreau, Journals *Winter*, Dec. 29, 1856

Daily outdoor activity is not a luxury to be enjoyed only on vacation or when you (finally) retire. It is not an overstatement to say that if you treat daily outdoor activity as a necessity rather than as a luxury it will change your life. Make yourself a priority. Women especially seem programmed to take care of everyone except themselves. They are easily co-opted into doing more work than they should and getting less recognition than they deserve.

I was recently talking to a group of young women lawyers who were having to work extra because they weren't getting the support they needed to do their jobs. I told them that they weren't going to get any extra points for suffering in silence. I told them, "This is business, not the f*ing red cross."

If that had been the end of the matter I wouldn't even be relating this story, but it was not. I didn't see this as a controversial statement – colorfully put perhaps (I am a trial lawyer after all!) – but in substance pretty obvious. It clearly was not obvious, however, to the young women with whom I was speaking or to their friends and even family members who were quickly quoting and spreading the advice. I recently met the mother of one of the women who had been there that day and upon meeting me she said, "Oh yes, the red cross!" There is something going on here and its not limited to work and office.

For those who cannot be persuaded to lay aside the burdens of others, let me put it another way. Assume life is like an airplane ride. In case of sudden loss of cabin pressure an oxygen mask will appear over your head. *Secure your own oxygen mask before attempting to help others.* Your daily escape out of doors is your oxygen mask. If you don't reach for yours, you won't be strong enough or last long enough to be any good to anyone else.

This is true for the truly burdened, not just those who are pressed for time. I have a cousin who has raised a physically handicapped child while caring for a husband who is also confined to a wheelchair. She has real challenges in her life and it shows. Recently when I was talking to her on the telephone I told her she should play golf once a week. My cousin hasn't been active in years, but I remember that she was a good athlete as a child. Even though I don't play golf myself, I thought it would suit her as it does many people who have a natural albeit dormant athletic ability. And since you usually play with other people and it takes a certain amount of time to get around the course, I thought it would offer the support and structure she would need to get started and keep it up.

Well there was silence on the other end of the line. Here she is with faced with more that needs to be done than can ever be accomplished in the day and I was telling her to play golf. I'm sure she's been given lots of advice over the years, but I could tell this was a new one and I think she began to wonder if I were losing it. So I told her to run it by her daughter, who despite her physical handicap is completing college and applying to law school, and her husband, who despite his illness has made the family financially secure. I was pretty sure they would agree because, in many ways, both her husband and her daughter are more mentally and emotionally stable than she. They had no choice but to reach for their own oxygen masks. For some time now my cousin hasn't taken the time to reach for hers thinking she didn't need it like they did, but she was wrong, and it's not doing them or her any good. Even she is not the red cross and neither are you.

E.

Workweek and Travel

*The really efficient laborer will be found not
to crowd his day with work, but will saunter
to his task surrounded by a wide halo of ease
and leisure.*

– H.D. Thoreau, Journals *Early Spring*,
Mar. 31, 1842

During the week most of us need an efficient way
to work some outdoor time into our day, ideally everyday
but at least 3-4 out of 5 weekdays. Running has always been
my mainstay midweek activity. Since it's right outside the
door, it's quick and easy and I can do it in pretty much any
weather. If you're not a runner, you can almost always take a
brisk walk.

I travel *nowhere,* no matter for how short a time,
without my running shoes and clothes. I have jogged around

every major and minor city I've ever visited, and given that a
lot of those trips were for business, my morning run has
usually been my only "tour" of the locale. On more than one
tiresome trip, it has been the highlight of my day. I have
fond memories of the adobe architecture of Stanford
University in a morning fog, daffodils blooming in St. James
Park around Buckingham Palace and Central Park under a
blanket of fresh snow. I have no fond memories of spending
the rest of those days inside conference rooms!

Even midweek, I get to the barn two mornings a
week to ride my horse. Since I have to drive to the barn, this
takes more time, so two mornings a week I get in late. One
of the advantages of being a lawyer is flexibility. We bill our
time so, other than court appearances and meetings, it
doesn't matter if we do our work at 6 in the morning or 6 in
the evening as long as it gets done.

Depending on your circumstances, arriving late or
leaving early one or two days a week may be a way to enjoy
a bike ride or a swim in the local pond even midweek. How
many of us have left work early to watch or coach a kid's
game or attend a dentist or doctor's appointment? Daily
outdoor activity is by definition "personal time." Even
better, if you are able to telecommute one or two days a
week, you can use the time you would have spent
commuting to head outside. Particularly in the winter when

the days are short, working from home may enable you to get outside midday when the sun is at its highest. Your mood will get a lift too.

I live on lake that is bordered by a main road to town 12 miles away. Many evenings I see a man stop on his way home from work and swim the mile across the lake. I imagine that he washes off the cares of the day before he arrives in the door a happier, saner, less anxious person. Good for him (and his family!)

F.

Weekend

Nature, the earth herself, is the only panacea.

–   H.D. Thoreau, Journals *Autumn*, Sept. 24, 1858

On the weekend we have more time to do something other than just a quick run around the block, ideally something that gets us not just outside, but into nature, the woods, the beach, the mountains. But we still have lots to do, which is why I like activities that don't take all day, much less all weekend. A mountain climb is generally an all day affair with a long drive to the bottom in addition to the long climb to the top. But hiking need not be limited to "bagging peaks." One of my favorite hikes goes part way up the mountain behind our house to a great viewing point, but nowhere near the top. In the fall, we clear the trails as we go so there'll be no obstructions on that long down hill cross country ski run next winter. We typically do it Sunday morning and are home in time (and in appetite) for waffles and scrambled eggs. A two hour bike ride is also a favorite weekend trip.

Downhill skiing is fun and I make time for it a few times each winter, but not every weekend. With getting to the mountain, it takes at least all day and for many people all weekend. And considering the price of the lift ticket, it doesn't make much sense to leave after just an hour or two. So I am big fan of cross country skiing. I can do it very near home and it can't possibly take all day. In fact it's pretty hard to do it for much more than an hour or two if you're skiing up and down hills on wooded trails like I am. That leaves the rest of the day for grocery shopping or cooking dinner or anything else that needs doing.

Now mind you, you are not going to impress people with any of this and in our competitive world choosing to live a life that doesn't impress people takes a lot of fortitude (which is why, as obvious as this all is when you think about it, I have to write this book). When your friends are telling tall tales about their annual summer trip to scale the 3000 foot mountain a couple of states over, no one will be impressed with your regular Sunday morning hike before brunch. Same with your Saturday afternoon 15 mile bike ride, which will be easily topped by your coworker's once a year 100 mile "century" charity event. When your neighbors are bragging about their once or twice a winter weekend ski trips to the "big mountain" a long drive or airline trip away, no one will be impressed that you cross country skied in the woods near home practically every weekend that same winter.

But while they are climbing a big mountain, biking a hundred miles or taking a trip to a ski resort at most once a year, you will be hiking, biking, skiing and a variety of other things every weekend of the year. You'll feel good, look good, be happy and at the end of the day sleep like a baby – not just one week of the year while you're on vacation – but every single day. Come to think of it, that's pretty impressive!

11.

Let's Go Outside!

With those general principals in mind, we're ready to go outside. I've divided this list by seasons (for obvious reasons) but of course many (not all) of these activities can be enjoyed in a variety of seasons. I've combined the spring and the fall into one category, since many of the same activities are suitable for either of those shoulder seasons. Indeed, these are really three-season activities, although which three seasons depends on where you live. If you live in a cool climate, you will hike and bike spring, summer and fall; if you live in a warm climate, you will do those things fall, winter and spring. If you live somewhere in the middle, adjust accordingly. Once you begin to live more in tune with the seasons, eating, sleeping, working and playing with, rather than against, the earth's natural rhythm, your

Women at Play

activities, like your clothes and food, will naturally change throughout the year.

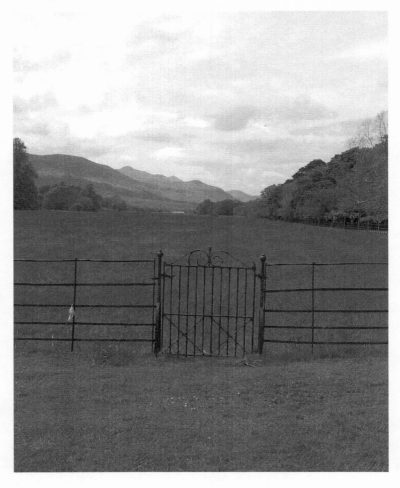

The view of the Reeks from Killarney House, Ireland

Spring / Fall

1. Running

As I have said at various points throughout this book, running is my mainstay outdoor physical activity all year round, especially midweek and while traveling when time is scarce. But that leaves the impression that running is a chore to be replaced by other, more enjoyable, activities when time permits, and while to some extent that's true, it's far from the whole story. I've listed running first, not simply because it's quick and easy, but because I realize that I love to do it and have relied on it more than any single other activity to keep me happy, healthy and sane.

There is something about running that is freer and more natural than just about any activity we do. Children love to run around and chase each other and invariably they're laughing when they're doing it. Not so long ago I realized that my favorite part of a lot of sports is the running part. I love running after the ball in soccer (even though I don't have much skill when I get it). I love running after the tennis ball on the tennis court. As I have said, maybe one reason I'm not a golfer is that there is no running involved.

When I had periods of very hard work studying engineering in college, my mother would ask me over the phone whether I had run that day. My mother is not an athlete so it struck me as odd that in the middle of studying for exams, she would be concerned about whether I was running. I realize now that she was asking the question, not because she is into running, she isn't, but to try to gauge just how bad things were. If I were getting the run in, things might be busy, but they were under control. There have been very few times in my life when I have not gotten it in.

I have been a runner for practically my entire life. When I was a kid, my father, who was a lifelong athlete, went to the local high school track to run a mile or two a couple of times a week. He took us and the next door neighbor kids with him and we knew that four times around the quarter mile track made a mile long before we learned fractions in school! I ran on the track and cross country teams in high school, beginning as one of two girls on the boys' teams since there were no girls' teams at the time. Our first coach, who was very supportive, had a healthy outlook. He said if we were still running in five years he would consider that he had been successful and he was.

All of that having been said, I was never a brilliant runner, and didn't run competitively in college. I did run regularly though, 4 miles a day, every day, no matter the weather. For most of my adult life, I have run about 3 (flat) miles a day, three or four times a week. I have never run a marathon or half marathon and never wanted to. I don't time myself, but I do try to be back in time for meetings, meals, etc.

Over the years, John and I have come up with a strategy for running together even though he is clearly much faster than I am. He just takes it easy (only kidding). What we do is we start out together at what for him is a slow jog. After about a mile, he goes ahead and runs fast, a half a mile out and a half a mile back to me. Then we run together for another mile. He does one more sprint out and back to me before we finish up together.

The result is that John has run a mile farther and substantially faster for 2 miles of the run than I have. It's a very healthy workout for him because he has a mile warm-up with me before he starts running fast and a similar cool down at the end. Equally beneficial, he gets in some speed work which most recreational runners, including me, neglect. (Yet another reason why it's a good idea to play other sports, such as soccer or tennis or tag with your kids, where you will naturally run at top speed to get what you're after. As with diet, variety is the natural way to get everything you need without even thinking about it.) This format can be varied to accommodate runners of many different strengths and abilities.

Many regular runners have to stop running at some point in their 30s and 40s due to injuries or simply wear and tear, particularly on the knees. For this reason alone, if you like to run and would like to keep running, it pays to run fewer miles. I ran every day in high school and college and through my early 20s. I was always prone to soreness in my knees and at some point cut back to running no more than every other day and generally no more than three times per week. John and I have stuck to this rule and we rarely run two days in a row.

You might ask, if running causes so much injury, why do it at all? In fact, you have to do high impact sports such as running to maintain bone strength and avoid diseases like osteoporosis. So again, in my opinion and without necessarily a scientific study to prove it, I say that moderation is key. It's important to continue to be able to include impact activities in your daily life so it's essential not to overdo it at any one time. (Actually I recently read about a study that concludes that running is good for your knees as long as you avoid injury – another benefit of moderation.)[6]

---

6. Gretchen Reynolds, "Phys Ed: Can Running Actually Help Your knees?", *New York Times*, Aug 11, 2009.

Since I was in high school, I, and various members of my family, have run a Thanksgiving Day road race. The race is one of the oldest in New England on a route marked out through the streets of a small Connecticut town. You know you're not in the Olympics when a 5 mile race is actually 4.7 miles because that's just the way the route came out. This is the only race that I run every year, and given that more than 10,000 people run it, for those of us well in the middle of the pack it's more of a social event than a race.

Still, it's something to gather with all of those people, many of whom do it every year just like we do, at the end of the calendar year and the start of the holiday season. You can't help but remember the many other years you've stood there – in the rain or snow or balmy Indian Summer weather – and as the years go by it's a thrill simply to be standing there yet again 12 months later. When someone asks me why I run relatively little, why I don't run more races or train harder, I jokingly say that I have only so many miles in me and I want them to last 'til I'm 95. But it's no joke. I have always done a variety of activities for enjoyment, but I also do it so that hopefully I will have a few more miles in me for many years to come.

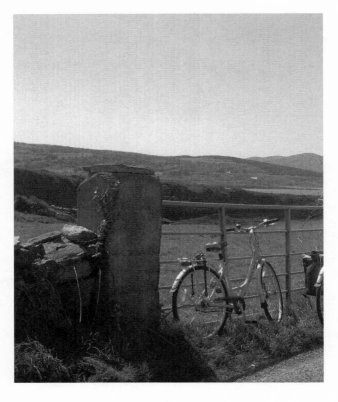

Sheep's Head, West Cork, Ireland

2. Bicycle Riding

Bicycle riding is so easy, so much fun and so accessible for most people that I am amazed that more adults don't do it regularly. Most of us rode bikes as kids and if you haven't done it in a while, it really does come back to you. Bicycle riding is a great activity to mix in with running or other high impact sports because it's easy on the joints such as knees which can suffer from too much running or the quick stop and go movements of a game like tennis. So why isn't everybody doing it?

I think the real problem is that bicycling, like a lot of simple activities that we all did as children, has been co-opted by the serious competitive types. When I say "bicycling" the word no doubt conjures up a spandex clad individual, neither male nor female, doubled over the handlebars of a racing bike and sporting plastic headgear complete with fins straight from my father's first car – a 1950s Chevrolet. When they gather in groups, these bicyclists look like an alien race from a Star Trek rerun.

There is little in this picture to which most reasonable people, particularly women, would aspire. Obviously there is something in this getup that appeals to some male concept of strength and power, otherwise I don't believe they'd be caught dead in it, but it escapes me, and most women rightly conclude that this look isn't going to do anything for them.

So let me begin by saying you don't need to look like this to go for a bike ride. Here, particularly, I think if you keep the image of Audrey Hepburn foremost in your mind, or even Paul Newman in the *"Raindrops Keep Falling on My Head"* scene from *Butch Cassidy and the Sundance Kid*, you will be more likely to see this as something you might like to do.

On a recent visit to Ireland, a few of my cousins, some of their kids and I cycled one morning a 12 mile route around the Lakes of Killarney in Killarney National Park. The views of the lakes with the Kerry mountains in the background make this a spectacular short bike ride. A stop for coffee at Dinis Cottage at the halfway point completes the idyll. After we finished, we ran into more cousins (men) who'd also been riding that morning, "training" for a 120 mile charity bike ride around the Ring of Kerry. They anxiously compared mileage and times and you can bet there was no stop for coffee at Dinis Cottage. If this sort of thing appeals to you, then by all means go for it. But if it doesn't, be assured that it's not the only way to enjoy a bike ride of a sunny Saturday morning in May.

a) the bike

First of all, ride a nice, comfortable upright bike. No one who is not in the Tour de France should be bent over a racing bike on a Sunday afternoon. Yes you will go slower on your upright bike. You will be less aerodynamically efficient. But where are you going in such a hurry? Nowhere!

Do not ride a mountain bike on paved roads or sidewalks. Those bikes with the little fat tires go too slowly and take too much effort to push on a paved surface. You want to feel like you are cruising along at a nice rate of speed. You want a bike with big wheels and mid size tires, neither the skinny tires of the racing bike nor the small, fat tires of the mountain bike.

I don't ride a mountain bike at all. All that bouncing around and popping over fallen logs looks a little ridiculous to me and not something that I'd like do on a bike. I realize that in certain parts of the country, particularly California, there are relatively smooth and well maintained off-road trails and therefore lots of mountain biking. We don't have a lot of that in New England, so it's not something with which I'm familiar. Here, unless you want to do a lot of bouncing around, you're better off sticking to paved roads.

For this purpose you want a bike that looks pretty much like an old-fashioned three-speed that your mother or grandmother rode in the 1930s, '40s or '50s, except that the bike you buy today is likely to have 18 or 21 gears which will make easy work of any hill. John collects or rather can't seem to turn down old Raleigh bicycles. I have a lovely cream-colored five-speed that I ride around the lake. I also bring it to Boston to ride up and down the Esplanade which is pretty flat. I generally prefer my 18 speed upright hybrid for really hilly terrain, but recently, when I lent that bike to a visiting niece and did a somewhat hilly ride with the Raleigh, I found that it worked better than I had expected. It's amazing how you get conditioned to the latest thing and forget that the previous latest thing worked pretty well too. I guess that's marketing!

If you haven't ridden a bike in a while and especially if 18 or 21 gears are new to you, take a little time to learn how to use them. This may sound obvious but on that ride around the Killarney Lakes, I noticed that one of my cousins was working much too hard, until I realized she wasn't using the gears. I promise you will consider it time well spent when you smoothly switch to a lower gear for that first uphill climb.

b) clothing, equipment

So now you have the bike and you're ready to jump on and go out for a ride. That's right, you don't need any specialized polyester clothing. I often wear cotton Capri pants when I'm riding my bike. The mid-calf length works really well because the pants don't get caught in the chain. In warmer weather, I wear cotton shorts. A T-shirt or sleeveless shirt works fine. If it's chilly or windy I carry a wool or cotton sweater and a windbreaker. I don't need Gortex, I'm not going anywhere in the rain and it doesn't have to be breathable. If it gets hot, I can take it off and this isn't Everest, a little sweat won't kill me.

Most of the time I wear a straw hat when I'm riding my bike. (I don't wear a helmet and, since I know that's controversial, I will address it separately below.) Obviously the hat must be chosen carefully. It must fit snugly enough not to blow off in the wind and have enough of a brim to keep the sun out of your eyes, but not so much as to catch the wind and blow off. Once you find it, you will get a lot of use out of this hat. You can wear it sailing, at the beach or out in the garden on a windy day.

All of my bike rides are day trips and most are for an hour or two in the morning or afternoon. I never do long-distance trips where I carry my own gear. I am not a pack horse and this goes doubly for hiking (more on that later). I do have a pannier on my bike in which to throw a spare sweater and windbreaker and oftentimes something for lunch or tea. Alternatively, I tie a bag or backpack onto the bicycle rack with a bungee cord. You absolutely need a bicycle rack on back of your bike. Baskets hanging off the handlebars are cute, but affect the steering when they get too heavy. Never, ever ride your bike with a backpack on your back. It will be uncomfortable and throw off your balance.

I do carry a water bottle in a holder attached to the frame of the bike, but I would never use one of those backpack water holders out of which you sip the water through a straw as you go. Again I don't want anything on my back, and I'm not in so much of a hurry that I can't stop and take a drink. On the contrary, stopping every now and then to admire the view or pick up something at a general store is part of the fun.

There is one thing I have picked up from the serious bicyclists that I like and for what it's worth will pass on. I have added toe clips to my pedals, sort of an open ended basket that holds your foot on the pedal. Technically, as I understand it, toe clips allow you to pull up on the pedal as well as push down on it as you're riding. Serious cyclists no longer use these toe clips as they now have special shoes that actually lock onto the pedal. I have never used those and am not sure they would be suitable for recreational cyclists as it would seem they might prevent you from getting your foot off the pedal if you needed to in an emergency. I do find toe clips comfortable, however, and miss them whenever I rent a bike without them. No one needs them to get started and you may decide never to bother with them at all, but if you become a regular recreational cyclist you might give them a try to see if you find them comfortable too.

c) helmets

I don't wear a helmet when I'm riding my bike. This is right up there with not owning a TV for raising eyebrows, but I grew up riding my bike without a helmet and it didn't seem to do me any harm. Helmets are not particularly comfortable and on a warm day they take away that "breeze through your hair feeling" that is half the fun of riding in a convertible, skiing down the hill or riding your bike.

I once saw a picture in the paper of Caroline Kennedy bicycling with her husband near their summer house in the Hamptons. They were both clad in regulation gear bent over the handlebars of their racing bikes, unrecognizable behind sunglasses and helmets. They looked like they were in a war zone. They did not look carefree. Here she is, one of the richest women in the world in one of the most beautiful summer places in America and she didn't look like she was having fun. Something is wrong with this picture. I asked myself, "Can it really be that bad or have we just convinced ourselves that it is and if so why?"

Helmets say that you are engaged in a dangerous activity or in a dangerous place or both. Now remember, this is a look competitive men like. They think it makes them look tough and manly and maybe it does, but I don't need to look tough or manly. Moreover, the fact that they are wearing helmets racing down major roadways at 50 miles per hour (engaging in dangerous activities, in dangerous places) doesn't necessarily mean I need to wear one riding on a quiet country road on Sunday morning.

At the other end of the spectrum, helmets may be a good idea for young children just learning to ride a bike, though everyone of my generation managed to learn how to ride a bike without one and I never heard of any kid being seriously injured while learning to ride a bike without a helmet. In any event, I am past that stage now.

Because I knew that this would be a controversial position, I took a look at the statistics. Not surprisingly, per mile, riding in a car is more dangerous than riding your bike and yet no one wears a helmet in the car. Tripping on stairs, steps or ramps is more likely to land you in the emergency room than any amount of bike riding. Most surprising to me, fully half of the deaths that occur to bicyclists occur at night. Ninety percent (90%) of all deaths are men. Lastly, one third of those deaths involved alcohol.[7] So I guess if you're a guy, out drinking and riding your bike at night you'd better wear a helmet. But for the rest of us, bicycle riding is no more dangerous than any other aspect of daily life and if we exercise some common sense as to where, when and how fast we ride, it can be a lot safer than most.

I wonder if this isn't another example of looking for a rule that will fix everything, "a law which we may obey." We like to think that if we just wear a helmet then we will be safe, no matter what. We don't have to slow down or watch where we're going, we just put on a helmet. We don't have to accept that our choices may be constrained, by overcrowded roadways and rush hour, we just put on a helmet. But the truth is that a helmet is no substitute for

7. 2005 Statistics from the Dept of Transportation-NHTSA

good judgment. Real outdoor activities, even everyday ordinary ones like riding a bike or sledding down the hill, are not amusement park rides. Life is not a no-risk proposition, and simply putting on a helmet cannot make it so.

I don't forgo a helmet simply because I'm too lazy to wear one. I am making a more affirmative statement than that. I want to say and stand for the proposition that life is not so bad, the world is not so dangerous and all our decision making need not be driven by fear. I want to look strong and healthy, upright and happy, not scared and defensive. It is the same statement I make when I ride around in my classic convertible that is far more open than even convertibles of today, the windshields and windows of which have crept up around the driver to protect him or her from the dangers of the road.

I protect myself from the dangers of the road by choosing when and where to drive. You won't see me in my roadster jostling with semi-trailers on interstate highways. You will see me on a quiet country road on a sunny Sunday afternoon traveling at a reasonable rate of speed – stone cold sober, both hands on the wheel, not talking on the phone, not drinking coffee and not putting on my makeup. I have the real security (not perfect security, nothing in real life is perfect) that comes with exercising good judgment. That makes a lot more sense to me than taking an unreasonable risk and pretending I've mitigated it to any significant extent by wearing a helmet.

I learned something else from the statistics; when people are required to wear helmets, many of those who would otherwise ride a bike simply give it up. It goes without saying that the benefits of bike riding far exceed the danger of riding without a helmet. So, for the time that I'm out there – driving my convertible, skiing downhill or riding my bike – I want to have fun, and look like I'm having fun, having entrusted my safety to the exercise of good judgment in deciding when, where and how to play.

d) where and when to ride

Depending on where you live, you will want to give some thought to when and where to ride your bike. When riding on the roads, it pays, for the sake of both safety and enjoyment, to figure out a route that keeps you off of the busiest ones. We always have at least a couple of routes of varying lengths that start and finish right at home. Once you have them figured out, it's easy to just jump on your bike when you have a free hour and go for a ride. It's worth putting in a little time up front to find quiet roads that keep you off your area's busiest thoroughfares.

Here is another area where you might borrow from your local cycling club. (I may not like their outfits, but I'm perfectly willing to borrow their suggestions if they're good ones.) In our area, the local cycling clubs have marked regular routes particularly on scenic roads. You might be able to find maps of the routes on the Internet, but you may also notice painted arrows on the roads themselves indicating where to turn. The best thing about these routes is that they often point out quiet and more scenic alternatives to busy highways. So if you see one of these arrows directing you off of the main road, you might follow it on your bike or in a car or at least pull out a map when you get home to see if it suggests a nice "detour" you might work into your own regular ride.

Time of day can also make a big difference. When we lived north of Boston, we loved riding our bikes up and down the scenic two-lane roads along the coast. Unfortunately, especially in the summer, everyone else enjoyed driving up and down the same roads in their cars, and as these were older roads without much shoulder, it got a little crowded.

We found that early on Saturday and Sunday mornings, even in the summer, we had the roads to ourselves. We devised a route from our house to a favorite breakfast place (I'm big on breakfast, especially after a morning hike or bike ride!) 10 miles away and had arrived back at home long before most people had finished their second cups of coffee and more importantly gotten into their cars. We've also found that late Sunday afternoons or evenings when the days are long can also be a quiet time on the roads and a great time to get out on your bike, maybe with a picnic supper to enjoy in some scenic spot along the way.

In addition to riding from home, we have also always enjoyed putting our bikes on the car and riding some route within a day's drive of where we live. We have several books of recommended bicycle routes in most of the New England states. Most of them have shorter or longer options within the same ride. This is a great way to get a change of scenery and add some variety to your bicycling. During the summer we choose a route with a swimming spot; we save certain rides for the fall when we know the foliage will be beautiful.

We also often rent bikes when we travel on vacation. All tourist destinations have bike rental shops and it's a great way to take in the scenery while shaking out the cobwebs after a plane trip or hotel stay. We don't do long-distance bike trips even with a van along to carry the gear. I suppose on vacation, as in life, I enjoy more variety than that. I don't really want to spend five or six straight days on a bicycle going 50 or even 30 miles a day. And if you do do one of those trips, you're committed to cycling even if the weather doesn't cooperate (and since Ireland is one of my vacation destinations, uncooperative weather is something with which I am familiar). But I love renting bikes on a warm sunny day and heading out for a spin through the countryside.

I suppose my first long cycles (15 or 20 miles) were in Ireland with my cousins when we were young teenagers. We rode whatever bikes we could find around the farms. They had hand brakes (unlike my bike at home) and three gears at the most, if we were lucky. One of our favorite routes was from home to Kenmare and then Killarney, two of the most scenic towns in Ireland. At about the halfway point we would stop at my cousin's Auntie Hannah's (on her other side) and she would give us fabulous tea and everything to go with it. I'm sure that Auntie Hannah, like all Irish people of her generation, had used a bike for basic transportation before everyone had cars. What she must have thought of three girls out for a big cycle I can only imagine, but I'm sure the "lunacy" was attributed, rightly, to the "Yank."

A couple of years ago John and I did the same ride on rented 21-speed hybrid road bikes. About halfway through, when John realized how long and hilly it was, he looked at me and said, "This is crazy!" I reminded him that my two (female) cousins and I had done the same ride when we were kids, on ill-fitting, one-speed bikes and hadn't thought that much of it. He cheered up when he realized that we'd finished the climb and the rest of the ride was all downhill.

e) riding with men

Bike riding is something that John and I have done together for as long as we've known each other. When I first met him, John was well on his way to becoming a serious spandex cyclist. Since even if I had wanted to become a serious cyclist (which I didn't) I never could have kept up with him, how have we managed for so long to ride together?

Initially, it didn't look too good. There was the first long trip we took together in college where John sprinted ahead of me up the hills of northwest Connecticut until he got so far ahead I simply got off my bike and sat down by the side of the road. So if John in front didn't work maybe we should try Joan in front. That was better in that I wasn't disheartened by seeing him so far ahead of me, but as John knew (although I didn't at the time), by being in front, I was doing the lion's share of the work, especially cycling into the wind, and John was essentially coasting behind me.

It was ultimately John who figured out the solution. He would ride in front of me, especially if there were any amount of wind, and I would ride right behind him "drafting" just like the best cyclists do in serious bike races. If, like most recreational bike riders, you've never experienced or thought about the effect of riding right behind someone while heading into the wind, you are in for a big surprise and a nice one if you're the person in back. It really is extraordinary how much less effort is required to go second.

Where riders are of equal strength, the usual strategy is to take turns being in front. But where one rider (say, for example, the husband) is much stronger than the other (say, for example, the wife) you simply leave the strong one in front most of the time. The result is that at the end of the ride, the stronger rider has had a good workout, but the weaker one is still standing, even though they've covered the exact same ground.

Of course it takes some skill to be the rider in front because that rider can't go too fast or the one behind will not be able to keep up and get the benefit of drafting. But if the one in front is such a serious competitive athlete, he should have some skill, right? This is a classic example of turning what at first seems like a problem to everyone's advantage, with the result that people of different abilities, which generally describes most families and friends, can play together.

John occasionally thinks a tandem bicycle would be the perfect solution, since then he could drag me along as fast as he wanted to go. We tried renting one once in Sanabel Island, Florida, a nice flat island good for biking. Initially, I tried riding in the front seat. To our surprise, that didn't work at all. We couldn't even keep the bike upright to get started. Apparently if you're riding a bicycle built for two and one person is much bigger and heavier than the other, the bigger and heavier person needs to go in front.

Once we figured that out and put John in front, things seem to go a lot better and we headed off for our ride. At the end of the day, John remarked that the whole thing was much more difficult than he'd expected and his muscles were tired even though the terrain was relatively flat. I said I'd had exactly the opposite reaction; the whole thing seemed dead easy to me. On reflection I realized that my only difficulty was that my feet couldn't keep up with the spinning pedals! I'm sure there must be some way to ride a bicycle built for two such that both riders are doing some of the work, but it may be that the riders need to be of relatively even strengths, or perhaps one needs a different kind of bike. For some reason we have not tried one since. Maybe if John finds a nice old tandem Raleigh . . .

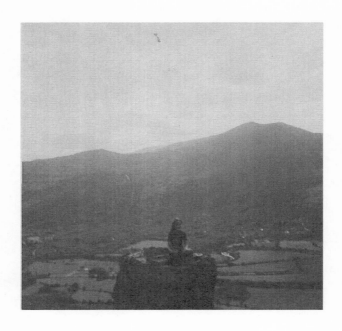

*The author atop the Two Stones,
County Kerry, Ireland, 1973*

3. Hiking

My first hikes were around my aunt's and uncle's farms in the mountains of County Kerry. My mother had three sisters living in Ireland, one stayed on the home farm and the other two married into neighboring farms, all around a 5 mile ring made by two roads in a river valley. The valley is surrounded by mountains covered with furze, ferns, heather and rocks, but no trees; there aren't a lot of trees in Ireland.

Behind one of the farms, up on the mountain ridge, there were two large boulders, no doubt left behind by some retreating glacier, that were visible from just about anywhere in the valley. They were known in the family as the Two Stones and the year that I was 11 my aunt promised that she would ask a couple of the older boys to take my cousin Mary and me up there. Well we didn't want to wait for the boys so Mary, who was 10, managed to find her way through the farm fields to the bottom of the mountain and from there we started working our way up.

Unfortunately, while the Two Stones are visible from just about anywhere in the valley, they are not visible once you actually start the climb. Still, there being no trees, this being an Irish mountain, we had lovely views of the three farms the whole way up and weren't all that worried about actually reaching the Two Stones. But thanks to Mary, who probably had been a good way up on more than one occasion collecting sheep, we did get there. We climbed up on top of the Two Stones and stood waving down to the valley below, too delighted with our accomplishment to worry that we might get in trouble. The farmers in the fields saw us, everyone came out of the houses to look up at us and we were famous before we ever made it home to tell of our exploits.

Right then I was hooked. For the next few years my cousins and I, on our own or with the help of like-minded adults, assaulted most of the peaks in the area including Carrauntoohill, the highest mountain in Ireland. It was a number of years later before I first did any real hiking in America when John was living in Vermont. I was not impressed. In Ireland, because there are no trees, you have excellent views during the entire climb. In New England, however, you hike up for two hours in the trees, get to the top, have a view and then turn around and spend two more hours in the trees going down.

I also found the hiking less interesting. In Ireland, at that time, most of the mountains we climbed had no marked paths. The farmer who went up there for sheep gave you directions or you read a guidebook that said something like "follow the stream up and careful you don't fall down the cliffs on the left" or you simply stood at the bottom and looked up. With experience you learned that what looked like a smooth grassy path from the bottom was in fact boggy and wet and that you'd be better off keeping to the rocky, if uneven, terrain where you'd stay dry (always an issue in Ireland). In New England, you followed marked and well worn paths, a necessity given the dense woods, but just not as interesting as trying to figure out the route yourself.

So over the years we've come up with a few strategies to make hiking more fun and interesting. Whenever possible, we hike ridge trails from which you get great views for more of the hike than just at the top. Or we choose trails that for whatever reason are less tree covered and, therefore, have better views. A lake or river provides a similar sense of openness. We also tend to hike in the spring and fall, when there are fewer leaves on the trees so that even if you don't have a view, you feel much less closed in (and there's an added bonus - no bugs!).

I especially enjoy getting off the marked paths. When we bought our house in New Hampshire, inside the broom closet tacked to the back of the door was a 50-year-old trail map of the hills around our house. We noticed that the map showed trails and old roads that were not shown on modern maps. We spent time looking at the map and consulting with the locals to see if we could figure out which unmarked trails or unused roads might still be accessible for hiking or cross country skiing. We followed one old road to a lovely site with a view and an orchard that once surrounded a house long since gone.

While these trails may not be as strenuous as a marked path up a 3000 foot mountain, there is a far greater sense of adventure when you're not exactly sure where you're going and don't know exactly what will be around the next corner or at the end when you finally get there. There is an irony to amusement park rides in that because you know you are safe, the ride must be that much faster or the drop that much steeper to seem at all exciting. It's amazing how little it takes to create excitement when you're on your own. Halfway up the trail leading to the old house site, a wooden sign is tacked onto a tree warning "Beware of cougar. He likes blueberries too." We have yet to see one, but that sign never fails to give me a chill.

We don't go on overnight backpacking trips. I'm not opposed to camping, just carrying hearth and home on my back. For that reason all of the overnight camping trips I have done have been by canoe. Since most of our hikes are for a couple of hours or at most a half day, we don't have to carry much. A sweater and a windbreaker (the same ones we bring on our bikes) are sufficient even on cooler fall days. I usually bring a small thermos of tea or coffee (an Irish trick) along with a muffin or lunch to have at our halfway point. No "camel pack" can compete with a hot cup of tea on a brisk fall day.

We also try to pay attention to bird songs and animal tracks as we go to see if we can understand something of the world around us. It's amazing how difficult it is. Turkey tracks are pretty easy to identify once you know what they look like and know that there aren't likely to be any other birds with such big feet in your area. But we can spend all kinds of time debating whether we are looking at fox or coyote or maybe even elusive bobcat tracks and never be sure even when we get home and consult the books.

Despite (or maybe because of) years of higher education, we are ignorant of the most basic facts of the world around us and of any species other than our own, but we are trying to remedy that. We can now reliably identify at least a couple of bird songs in the woods around our house and it's like having new friends and neighbors we had no idea were there. There may be a foot of snow on the ground, but if the black capped chickadee is singing his phoebe song, I know that spring is on the way.

I would guess that the vast majority of people who have traveled far and wide to exotic locales inhabited by exotic creatures can identify very few of the most common birds and animals living right around them at home. Do you know the song of a robin? With cars and airplanes we have gained a superficial knowledge of a wider world, but does that make up for a lack of a deep knowledge of home? I think not, which is in why everyday play, like everyday food, should be local.

It seems that this year everyone I know is going to Costa Rica. Recently, talking to a few friends planning their trips, John mentioned that last fall we had taken a vacation to the beach in Rhode Island about 90 miles away. An acute listener accused us of having taken a "low carbon vacation." He said we had probably seen all of the same birds last fall in Rhode Island that our neighbors would see this winter in Costa Rica! Think of your local morning or afternoon hike as a low carbon vacation.

> *Such is beauty ever, neither here nor there,*
> *now nor then, neither in Rome nor in Athens,*
> *but wherever there is a soul to admire. If I*
> *seek her elsewhere because I do not find her*
> *at home, my search will be a fruitless one.*

–   H.D. Thoreau, Journals *Winter,* Jan. 21, 1838

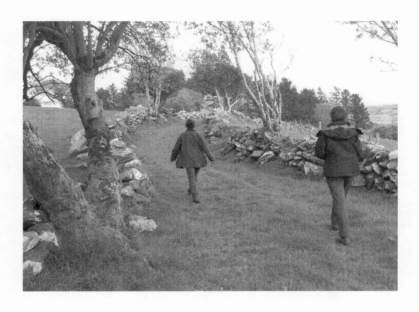

Walking in the Irish countryside

4. Walking

uitwaaien (Dutch)

- *literally "to walk in windy weather for fun,"*
- *figuratively "taking a short break in the countryside to clear one's head of day-to-day worries."*

- Adam Jacot De Boinod, *If you can't say it in English, just borrow,* Smithsonian, March 2006.

My mother is not an athlete, but she has always been a walker. Although she walked many evenings in fine weather, she was most tempted by a blowy, rainy day after the heaviest downpours had passed. Maybe it reminded her of home.

In Ireland this past summer it rained (and on many days poured) for 74 straight days from June to September. The previous summer was not a whole lot drier. More than cold or snow or blazing heat, rain is a challenge to regular outdoor exercise. In conditions like these, or anytime you have a stretch of wet weather, walking may be the best, if not only, option for exercise outdoors.

There is something forbidden, even dangerous, about venturing outside in bad weather, even if you are just walking around the block and are perfectly safe. If you're dressed properly, it's fun as well as exciting (see quote) and you can't help feeling that you're getting away with something. To be outside and comfortable in that kind of weather is like stealing home (or at least second).

But unless you live in the tropics, you'll need appropriate attire. Most importantly, you'll need a hat. This might not be the first thing that comes to mind for being outside in the rain, but it is among the most critical. I didn't realize this until I started riding a horse. You simply can't walk around a barn with an umbrella. It isn't done. (Apparently, and completely to my surprise, Sir Edmund Hillary brought an umbrella up Everest, but then he also had Sherpas!) So what you need is a hat with a brim, preferably a brim all around, not just in front like a baseball cap. It's amazing how vulnerable you feel if your head is getting wet (even if you're wearing a coat) and how comfortable you feel if your head is protected. Note, this is equally true in the grocery store parking lot.

Then of course you need a jacket or coat and, if it's really pelting and not likely to dry off anytime soon, rain pants. Most of the time I get by with a waxed cotton jacket and waxed hat. I also have waterproof rain gear, top and bottom, which I bought for hill walking in Ireland where you can get a drenching shower in the middle of an otherwise fine day. It's inexpensive and not breathable. It's just meant to keep out the water. Since I am not out for days at a time, I don't have to worry about hypothermia if I sweat a little on my way home.

To be clear, when I talk about walking I am not talking about parking your car at the far end of the grocery store lot so you can spend your precious free time crossing an asphalt wasteland dodging SUVs. I'm not talking about wearing a pedometer to record every routine step of the day. Nor am I talking about a once a year charity fund raiser. You can and should walk without a cause.

I am talking about selecting a few good outdoor routes near home that will give you exercise and fresh air in any weather. Your routes can be different lengths and varying terrain depending on the time and energy you have available. It's best to have at least one or two you can do right from home. Even a walk you've done a hundred times will be new and different on a blowy day or a moonlit winter evening.

I walk briskly, but I don't "speed walk." Speed walkers always look stressed out to me, like a horse trotting too fast that would be much more comfortable if he simply broke into the cantor. Nor do I carry weights and pump my arms artificially. I'm always a little afraid that swinging around dead weight will pull something that I'd rather not pull. And let's face it, it's just not elegant! In fact, I don't like to carry anything at all when I'm walking, even water. Unless you're walking at midday in Nevada in the summertime (not a good idea), if you're just walking 3 or 4 miles around home, you won't get dehydrated before you get back and you don't want to be carrying anything that interferes with swinging your arms freely as you go.

I have read that some yoga instructors have started giving "walking lessons" to teach people how to walk with correct posture. I'm in favor of anything that improves posture and it certainly makes sense that you should stand up straight, with your head up and shoulders back, when you're walking. You also don't want to be carrying anything (weights or water) that throws off your natural balance. I have an elderly cousin who always admonishes herself and her friends to stand up straight and she offers an excellent justification: bending over doesn't help!

I do walk at night especially in really hot weather or in late fall and early winter when the days are short. Once you get out there, most nights are not as dark as they seem from inside. Even if there are no overhead streetlights, your eyes adjust and after a while you can see quite well. This is well known to sailors who use red colored flashlights so as not to lose their night vision when they turn them on. Walkers, like sailors, should pay attention to the moon. I went out for a walk at night recently and with the full moon it was nearly as bright as day.

Since we don't have sidewalks or street lights, we bring a flashlight with us if we are out walking after dark. This is not so much to help us see, but to help cars see us if they are passing by. So unless there's a car coming, the flashlight is off. If you've been sitting at a desk all day, the early evening may be your only chance to get outdoors, and if you plan correctly, it can be a safe and refreshing end to the day.

If you're lucky, you may be able to incorporate a walk into your commute to and from work. For about 10 years, while I worked as a lawyer in downtown Boston, I commuted by train and had a brisk 15 minute walk from the station to the office. I walked no matter what the weather. Some days it gave me an extra 30 minutes of outdoor exercise in addition to my regular run and other days it was my only outdoor time. In either case, you couldn't have paid me to give up the fresh air of my walk for a seat on a stuffy unreliable trolley, though many of my coworkers did and then complained when they couldn't find time to go to the gym!

John and I are now able to work from home for a part of each week, a huge help in incorporating everyday outdoor activity into our lives. But that doesn't mean we've given up our walk to work. On the contrary, on those days we head out the door and down the road, turn around and walk back and "arrive" at work refreshed and ready for the day. If any of your regular destinations are within walking distance, leave your car at home and enjoy the journey. We regularly walk to our local library, a distance of about a mile away.

Walking, more than anything else, is the perfect everyday outdoor activity. You can do it in any weather, anywhere, and for as long or short a time as you like. You can take a walk as a relaxing coda to an active outdoor day or as your only outdoor activity after a day at the office. It can be the least strenuous or the most strenuous thing that you do, and either way, it's worth doing. Our neighbors are always surprised to see us out walking, since they know that we do lots of vigorous outdoor activities, including running. I find that a good walk shakes out muscles that have gotten stiff from a long bike ride or a day of skiing. If I've been inside for a few hours, there's nothing like a brisk walk in the fresh air "to clear one's head of the day's worries." If it's raining, a walk may be the only option. I was talking to my mother recently about growing up in Ireland with so much rain and she said, "Oh, but the rain was different there. You just went out in it."

> *He whom the weather disappoints,*
> *disappoints himself.*
>> — H.D. Thoreau, Journals *Winter,*
>> Jan. 26, 1852

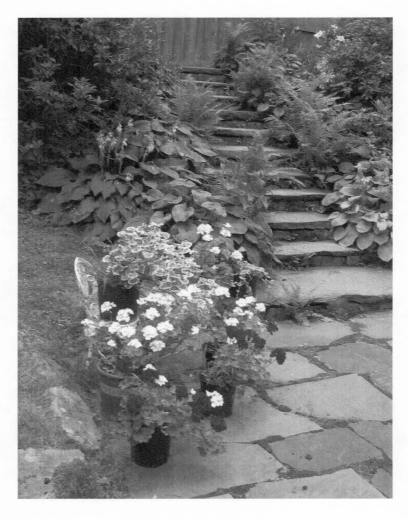

New Hampshire Garden

5. Work Out(side)

The previous owners of our house in New Hampshire were avid landscapers and gardeners. The woman of the house made a particular specialty of daffodils. She and her friend next door started the local Daffodil Festival and one of them was sure to come home with the top prize each year. Given the lateness of spring in the mountains of New Hampshire, it's not surprising that the appearance of the season's first flowers is an occasion for celebration. So every year around about April, John and I head out to the yard with rakes to carefully remove the blanket of matted leaves concealing literally thousands of daffodils ready to announce the start of a new growing year.

Fall and spring lend themselves to working outside. For several weeks each fall we rake the leaves (lots and lots of leaves) and in the spring we "thatch" the lawn with those same rakes (and free the daffodils). It's a big project that takes several hours each weekend for several weeks in a row and we love it. With the snow finally melted and the early spring sun streaming through the leafless trees, we can't wait to get out in the yard and give the grass a good scratch to clean up after the burrowing creatures or just to encourage the new green grass to grow. You will also see us outside putting the garden to bed and battening down the hatches for winter on an Indian Summer day when the leaves have turned brilliant colors transforming the waning autumn light to high noon.

Nowadays yard work and similar chores are done by "the man." You know, "the man" who comes to mow the lawn or clean the pool or deliver next year's firewood. But is all that convenience such a good thing? Some time ago, as my parents were waiting for "the man" to come rake their leaves, I took my two nieces outside and we all raked the lawn. The four-year-old especially dug right into it and wouldn't stop until we had all the leaves on the front lawn set out by the side of the road.

Kids like to be active and they like to accomplish things. Adults do too. I recently saw an article noting that with work becoming increasingly piecemeal and abstract, there is little satisfaction in having accomplished something by the end of the day. The writer opined that maybe that's why so many people can be seen at the Home Depot on the weekend – to do a job where they can see results.

Outdoor work, whether raking, gardening, snow shoveling or even washing the car, offers the same sense of satisfaction with the added benefit of enjoying the outdoors while you're at it. Since the nature of the work is always determined by the season and the weather, there is a connection to the natural world from working outdoors that you don't get from an indoor project. As Thoreau famously noted, chopping firewood warms you twice, once when you chop it and again when you burn it. We feel a particular connection to the wood in our wood stove this year. It came from a large oak tree that fell across the road in last year's ice storm leaving us without power for two weeks. As John says, that tree kept us cold for two weeks last year, but it will keep us warmer for a lot longer this year.

There is also something to be said for strengthening and suppling the body through natural activities. My cousins who are farmers in Ireland need no gym memberships to keep fit. The toned upper bodies of women riders are due as much to working around the barn as riding the horse. A carpenter who's strong from physical work even looks different from an artificially toned gym rat. Ironically we may have grown so used to admiring the one that we fail to appreciate the other, but I think there's something to be said for strength that is useful and not merely decorative.

And the best part about seasonal, outdoor chores? They end! The last leaf finally falls and gets raked into its pile (or the snow falls and the rest of the raking must wait until the spring). Daffodil season comes and goes like clockwork every year and we all move on to something else. So get out there and enjoy it while you can.

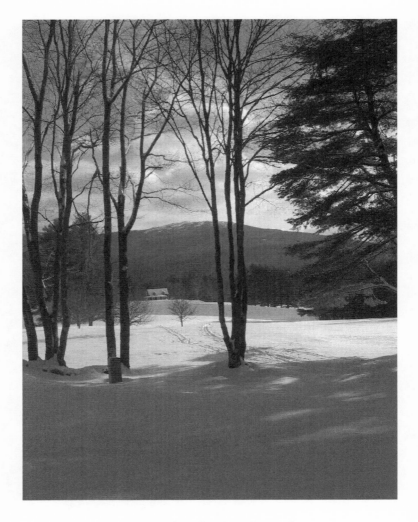

Mt. Monadnock, New Hampshire

Winter

Let us sing winter.

– H.D. Thoreau, Journals *Winter,* Jan. 30, 1854

Winter outdoor activities, perhaps more than those of any other season, remain true to the spirit of childhood play. Maybe it's because few of us grow up playing winter sports competitively. Skiing, ice skating and sledding were done just for fun and when conditions allowed. Certainly in New England, the transience of the right conditions is a big part of the excitement; you can only go sledding when it snows, you can't go ice skating unless it's been good and cold for a while, and any given day might be the last of the season.

I love winter in New England. I have no desire to escape to a warmer climate. I find "Florida" in a sunny southern exposure in the middle of a cross country ski trip or in the sun blazing on my back while I'm ice skating on the frozen lake. True, it only lasts for a short time in the middle of the day, but it's enough, as Thoreau says of the south wind, "to melt my soul."

Florida is sunshine and warm temperatures. But think about it, there isn't much that's brighter than the midday sun on a snow-covered landscape. Just read Sir Edmund Hillary's description of the blazing heat and blinding sun on clear days climbing Mount Everest.

So that leaves temperature. Yes, winter in northern states is cold, but that doesn't mean you have to be. Everyone knows that exercise raises your spirits, but no one really knows exactly how or why. One study speculated that by raising our internal body temperature, exercise improved our overall outlook. I think that has to be the case in the winter. No matter how warmly I'm dressed or how warm the room, I seem to get chilled after too long a time sitting inside. The colder I get, the less I want, or feel able, to do. I simply shut down.

Going outside in the cold and doing something active, on the other hand, has exactly the opposite effect. As long as you're properly dressed (more about that below) and doing something vigorous, you warm up pretty quickly. The warmer you get, the freer you feel and more equal to the tasks before you. The world is no longer a cold forbidding place. The temperature outside hasn't changed. You have changed by physically engaging with, rather than hiding from, the natural world. But the result is profound. "The cold is merely superficial. It is summer still at the core."[8]

---

8. H.D. Thoreau, Journals *Winter* Jan.12, 1855.

1. Winter clothing

There is no bad weather, just bad clothing.

Most people who say they hate the winter simply aren't dressed for it. This does not apply only to those who live where winters are snowy and really cold. Even if it rarely or never snows where you live, chances are temperatures do drop enough to make just going outside for a walk uninviting, unless you're dressed correctly. In this case, clothes really do make the woman or at least her outlook on the world.

T-shirts are not winter clothes. If you spend the winter wearing the same clothes you wear in the summer your home/office/car are overheated. It's actually a lot easier to dress properly for the winter if indoor spaces are kept cool. If your house is not overheated, you'll already be wearing long underwear under pants, shirt and sweater when you add the jacket, hat and mittens to go outside. If your house is it at 70°F, however, you'd have to change completely to be properly dressed to go outdoors on a winter day. Instead, most of us simply throw a winter jacket over the light pants and shirt we're already wearing and end up freezing when we go outside.

A typical complaint of proper winter clothing is that it's heavy or bulky. In fact, if you feel that way, you're wearing the wrong clothes for the environment. I'm a small person and can easily be overwhelmed by a lot of clothing. But in my experience, no matter how much clothing you have on, if it's the right clothing for the environment, it will feel, not only comfortable, but light. Conversely, no matter how little clothing you have on, if it's too hot out, you will feel weighed down. Much of the best winter clothing is thin and lightweight, think silk long underwear or a cashmere sweater. But no matter how much of it you have on, if you're wearing the right clothing on a cold day, it will feel light and comfortable (and you will feel strong and free) when you go outdoors.

Dressing for cold weather is actually pretty simple and whether you're wearing street clothes or clothes for more strenuous activity, the principles are the same. There is the inner layer (long underwear), the middle layers (a shirt and sweater) and the outer layer (a jacket). If you're wearing street clothes in the wintertime, the inner layer might be silk long underwear, the middle layers might be a cotton turtleneck and wool sweater and the outer layer a coat or jacket. Generally, the coat or jacket needs to be windproof to be effective.

Practically no one these days wears long underwear under their street clothes when they're doing routine errands like grocery shopping or buying gas, but we would all be a lot more comfortable on very cold winter days if we did. For women, silk long underwear is fantastic because it fits so easily under any clothes, even suits and dresses we wear to the office. I wear a sleeveless V-neck silk T-shirt almost every day from late fall to early spring. If you've never worn silk bottoms under your pants in the wintertime, you will be amazed at the difference they make carrying groceries through a cold parking lot. It's best if you wear them under pants that are somewhat loose (i.e. not your tightest jeans). It's more comfortable and the layers of warm air that build up between the loose layers of clothing really keep you warm. Add a wool sweater and a warm windproof jacket and you're ready for anything, from a trip to the post office to a good long walk.

The middle layers – a cotton turtleneck and wool sweater – shouldn't require much explaining, but like Katie Couric's turkey sandwich, maybe they do. When it's cold you'll want to cover your neck either with a cotton turtleneck or with a scarf. No matter how many clothes you're wearing, if you have an open collared shirt leaving your neck exposed, you will feel cold. Recently, as a change from turtlenecks, I started wearing silk scarves wrapped tightly around my neck with an open collared shirt or T-shirt under a sweater. It makes a nice change, and unlike the turtleneck shirt, if you do get warm, you can loosen the scarf or take it off altogether. Oh, and by the way, it looks good!

As long as you're not doing strenuous activity the turtleneck can be cotton, but in the wintertime the sweater should not be. There is no warmth in a cotton sweater. Again, if you go through the winter wearing T-shirts and cotton sweaters, your house is overheated and you are probably miserable when you go outside. A winter sweater needs to be wool. It can also be cashmere if you want to spend the extra money, but for everyday, wool wears better. You can also wear a synthetic fleece, but wool actually works better at wicking moisture away from your body and I think it feels warmer.

In recent years, when athletic winter clothing was largely taken over by synthetics, I remained a fan of wool and stuck to my wool sweaters and wool socks in winter. A couple of years ago, my confidence in wool was vindicated when long underwear made from very fine merino wool finally became available in skiing and sports shops. I now wear my merino wool long underwear on the coldest cross country ski days or to the barn riding my horse in the winter. It's so warm and comfortable that I wear only my heavy wool sweater over it when I go out for a ski. Since the shirt is not a turtleneck, to keep my neck warm and to protect it from the coarse wool of the heavy sweater, I wear an old silk scarf tied around my neck, which again I can loosen or take off when I warm up. I am neither a spandex cyclist nor a spandex skier!

To hear people tell it, like all allergies these days, allergy to wool is an epidemic. But I think the itchiness people attribute to wool is not due to allergies but to wearing it improperly in overheated environments. If you wear a wool sweater over a cotton turtleneck in a 60°F house my guess is you will not be itchy. Conversely, if you wear a wool sweater on a 70°F day you may well be itchy and it will have nothing to do with an allergy. In fact, I think there are synthetics in wool blends that cause more discomfort than pure wool in any environment. I have wool blankets on all of the beds in my house in New Hampshire and as long as the bedroom is not overheated – and it's not – no one is itchy. Indeed, the nights in New Hampshire are so cool that we use light wool blankets on the beds all year round.

On the other hand, while wool is great as an inner or middle layer, it's not enough as an outer layer in really cold climates. The outer layer doesn't need to be warm, as much as windproof. In fact the outer layer can be nothing more than a windproof shell, provided you're wearing enough underneath. For this reason wool coats, which are great in the spring and fall, are not enough as an outer layer in the wintertime in really cold climates such as the Northeast. If you don't believe me, just look at the faces of the people heading to their offices in Boston, New York or Chicago on a cold and windy January morning clad only in their wool coats.

I didn't really appreciate the importance of the windproof outer layer until just recently when I bought a mid-length insulated leather jacket. To my surprise, the jacket was much warmer than a thicker wool coat because the leather is windproof. I shouldn't have been so surprised since I have always appreciated my suede riding chaps on cold winter days and as a result even bought a pair of lined suede jeans for everyday winter wear. On really cold days, however, my outer layer of choice for getting to and from the office is a medium length mink coat that I got for practically nothing on eBay. It's warm and windproof and amazingly light and no down coat ever got as many compliments. (When it comes to dressing for the cold, the Russians know a thing or two.)

Finally, there is the issue of shoes. Years ago when I first started practicing law, I had to go to court on a very cold winter morning. I was wearing the uniform of the day, a skirt suit, nylons and pumps, and even though I was wearing a warm winter coat, the nylons and pumps just weren't cutting it on the walk from the office to the courthouse. My feet and legs were so cold that I had to duck into office buildings on the way to warm up. At one point, I seriously questioned whether I would be able to make it! Shortly thereafter, I gave up the pumps and bought a discrete pair of black lace up cowboy boots (at the time they were the only boots I could find) that I could wear under long skirts and pants to get around Boston. Fortunately, boots are in style now, from dress boots suitable for the courtroom to shearling ones for outdoor wear. So now, whether we're dressed up or dressed down, we can wear a comfortable pair of boots that will keep us warm no matter the temperature outside. I shutter (and shiver!) to think what we'll do when boots (not to mention trouser suits) go out of style.

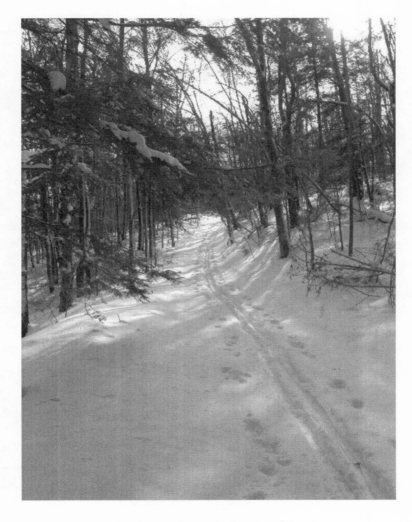

Skiing through the woods

2. Cross country skiing

Assuming we get the snow, as we did this year when the yard was snow covered from December 3 to April 12, cross country skiing becomes my mainstay outdoor activity for the winter. I still run when I'm in the city or when traveling, but whenever possible I cross country ski instead. It's a great break from running for the sake of one's knees and seems to involve a whole different set of muscles, but is equally aerobic.

More than that, cross country skiing, especially if you include some hills, is just plain fun. There's something about sliding along the snow and trying to keep your balance (not always successfully) that is a lot like the games you played as a kid. And because the hills are small and the skis are a bit unstable, and you're not cold and windblown at the top of some big mountain, the whole thing seems less serious than downhill skiing.

Let me begin by pointing out that I never ski golf courses as I find them really boring (for skiing, sledding is another story). I think that's worth noting at the outset because, for many people new to the sport, the golf course seems the obvious place to begin. Unfortunately, however, because it's so dull, it's an equally obvious place to end, and many people never find out how much fun cross country skiing can actually be. Even though many golf courses are hilly, they are simply too open to be interesting. There's no anticipating what's around the corner – there's no corner to go around and if there is you can already see what's around it. Also, because the area is so wide you don't feel like you're moving as much as you do going the very same speed on a narrower wooded trail. Golf courses are also less protected from the wind than trails in the woods. Cross country skiing on a golf course is like canoeing upwind across a lake – not nearly as much fun as paddling down a narrow, winding river.

John and I own our own cross country skis (they're not that expensive and given how often we use them owning is very quickly cheaper than renting). We also tend to cross country ski on our local hiking trails rather than at cross country ski centers that rent equipment and groom trails. We have "back country" cross country skis which are much less extreme than they sound. In fact, I recommend them for everyone except those who are going to ski only in parallel tracks set down by a machine or who are doing competitive skating style cross country skiing (neither of which I recommend). Back country cross country skis are a bit wider and shorter than traditional Nordic skis making them easier to turn as you ski down a narrow path in the woods. They also have metal edges, again to help with turning.

Even so, compared with downhill ski equipment, one has very little ability to control speed and turning on a downhill cross county run. So if you can't control yourself or the skis, you have to control the terrain by choosing the right trails for the right conditions. I am reminded of my physical chemistry professor freshman year at Yale who, when asked how he could get the class to pass without a curve, said with his Texas drawl, "I artfully write the test."

When picking a cross country ski route it pays to artfully write the test. We have several routes right in our area each of which has terrain of varying difficulty and steepness. When there is a lot of new deep snow or if the snow is a bit wet or sticky, you need the steepest trail possible to get going at all on the way down. When the snow is packed down, however, or if it's a bit slick, you will find yourself speeding down even the gentlest slope and the steep trails are unskiiable. The key is choosing the right trail on the right day.

The answer is not trading in your skis for snow shoes! I find it deeply concerning that so many relatively young, healthy even athletic adults give up cross country skiing in favor of snowshoeing because they are afraid of falling. Snow shoes are great for accessing trails that are simply too steep to ski, but if you're using them on gentle or even flat terrain simply because you're afraid of losing your balance, that's a problem. Keeping your balance keeps you young, and it's a case of use it or lose it. If you're used to recovering from a boggle on a ski trail, you will be able to recover from a trip on a sidewalk and you won't be so afraid of either. Contrary to what appears to be popular belief, there is no expiration date on balance. I was recently stunned to learn that a couple in our local ski group are in their 80s! They are healthy and active and like to have fun and their willingness to ski – and keep their balance – makes them seem young.

Because we ski on local hiking trails, we generally have to make our own tracks. Especially after a heavy snowfall, breaking trail can be hard work. But that's OK, we like the exercise and we're not looking for an amusement park ride. One weekend, when there was a particularly heavy snowfall, it took us three trips out to put down a trail on one of our regular routes. Each time we went out we did as much as we could and then turned around and enjoyed sliding home on the trail we had just made.

This is another great time to have a big strong competitive friend or husband. Simply put him in front and you can ski along behind batting cleanup. I occasionally take a spell out in front, but in truth John breaks a lot more of the trail than I do, which is fine since he's bigger and stronger than I am. At the end of our ski, we have both earned our hot chocolates.

Of course, if the snow has gotten crusty you may not be able to ski at all unless you find trails that are also frequented by snowmobiles which chop up the ice and in essence "groom" the trails. Only one of our local trails permits snowmobiles and we think that there is basically one guy who lives nearby who uses them. We have to ski a little way in from the road to get to the portion of the trail he uses and we are furious if it's past noon on Saturday and he has yet to come out and break up the trail!

There's something more to skiing local trails, breaking the trail yourself, than just great exercise. That weekend it took us three trips to break the whole trail we had fun! There's something adventurous – and active – about being the first to head into the woods after a big storm that is missing from the all inclusive – and passive – resort experience. It's satisfying to blaze the trail, essentially making your own fun. Before ski resorts built terrain parks, I used to be amazed at how long and hard snowboarders would work to build their jumps. I now think that for them there was both physical and mental satisfaction to designing and building the "question" before getting on the snowboard to execute an elegant (hopefully) ride in "answer." Few snowboarders (still in one piece) need to be reminded to artfully write the test!

Now I know there are more than a few die-hard downhill skiers out there (and I know a few) who can't imagine why anyone would want to waste their time cross country skiing, particularly to climb up a relatively small hill for a relatively short run down as compared with alpine skiing at a local resort. I'll have more to say about downhill skiing later, but there are a few obvious advantages to cross country skiing which downhill enthusiasts simply miss. First, you don't need a mountain to do it, so for many of us that means you can do it close to home. I have spent many happy hours cross country skiing in the state parks and nature preserves in the suburbs north and south of Boston and pretty much anywhere they get snow you can find trails to ski. Since it doesn't take all day and the trails are local, you can go out for a ski in the morning or afternoon and still have the rest of the day to get other things done.

Second, particularly in New England, there are a lot of days when you can happily cross country ski but would be miserable at a downhill resort. When it's very cold and windy, downhill skiing just isn't fun and sitting on the chairlift even less so. But you can cross country ski on wooded trails on even the coldest days in January and

February and be perfectly comfortable, indeed shedding layers as you go.

Third, because you have to work for that downhill run, haul yourself up the hill before you get to ski down it, you get far better exercise cross country skiing than you do riding a chairlift at the alpine resort (and in a much shorter amount of time).

A friend recently complained that the problem with skiing or sledding is that here in New England at least, you hardly ever get perfect conditions. Not true – the conditions are always perfect for something, you just have to figure out what. Like any activity you do on your own rather than at a resort, cross country skiing your local trails requires you to know the terrain and pay attention to the conditions. You can't simply assume that snow has been made even if none has fallen or that all trails are flat and smooth. Indeed the very same trail may be a green circle one day and a black diamond the next. But that is also its advantage. While one can quickly get bored of the perfectly groomed trails at a regular ski resort (and hence have to seek out ever steeper terrain usually miles from home), with ever changing conditions, a very few local trails can provide nearly an infinite variety of terrain and skiing experience over the course of a winter.

Like all natural outdoor activities, cross country skiing your local trails gives you a reason to notice what's going on in the natural world around you and a reason to care. When a degree above or below freezing makes the difference between sliding smoothly over the frozen snow and sticking in snow that has turned to concrete, you will know the temperature and which trails are likely to be sunny or shady at any point in the day. Most importantly, when development of yet another strip mall threatens your local trails, you will care, not just about an abstract political issue or some other species' habitat, but about a critical part of your habitat as an active member of the natural world.

Yes skiing local trails takes more effort than simply going to a resort and letting someone else do all the thinking, but I have found over the years, skiing, hiking, sailing, canoeing and horseback riding to name just a few, that having to figure out a few things for myself is actually more interesting and more fun. And the more I have to figure things out for myself, the less extreme the terrain needs to be to keep me interested and the less far afield I have to go to have a great time. Why limit yourself to answering someone else's question when you can double the fun by taking a hand in artfully writing the test?

3. Downhill Skiing

Go skiing when it snows. It would seem to go without saying that since outdoor activities are weather dependent, you should check the weather before deciding what to do on any given day. In fact, however, in our over-scheduled and time-pressed society, that basic principle is violated more often than not by weekend warriors trying to fit in outdoor pursuits around the constraints of work and other obligations. The one essential difference between sailors who have taken six months or a year to go cruising and the typical weekend sailor is not knowledge or experience. It's that the long distance cruiser can and does wait for the right weather in which to make the next leg of his cruise, while the weekend sailor goes out in marginal if not downright inclement weather because he has to be in the office on Monday morning.

Ireland has been a tourist destination for centuries and the Irish are well used to visitors short on time trying to take it all in. The Dingle Peninsula in County Kerry is a particularly scenic area along Ireland's southwest coast. The highlight of the coast road drive is the view at Slea Head out to the rocky Blasket Islands. The problem with touring

Dingle, however, is that more often than not the whole thing is covered in fog and there's nothing to see. As my Uncle Timmy would say, with typical understatement, "You want the day for Dingle."

Downhill skiing may well be the Dingle of outdoor winter sports. Because you are high on a mountain, everything – cold, wind, snow and ice – is more extreme. A cold or windy day at home may be a bitter day on the mountain and the lifts to the top may not even be open. For years, John has picked our downhill ski days based on the weather report, scheduling other less weather dependent activities around the ski days, rather than vice versa. If they are calling for highs in the teens and 20 mph winds, it's not a downhill ski day. Part of the fun of downhill skiing is going fast and that's a lot more fun on a sunny 30° day. As a result, in New England, March is a great time to downhill ski. The days are longer, the sun is higher in the sky and the temperatures are generally higher too. We have found that early spring is a great time to take a trip to the mountains as a still-snowy mountain in late March or early April easily beats a day of mud season at home.

If you pick the right day, you can enjoy the weather rather than huddling inside clothes, goggles and headgear fleeing from it. Recently I saw a classic ski poster hanging in a gallery window. It looked so appealing I stopped to try to figure out why. The two skiers were bareheaded except for goggles and sunglasses and wore slim ski pants and wool sweaters. They were enjoying rather than shrinking from the elements. Obviously, they had picked a nice day to ski. There may be more of them in Colorado than in New England, but all the more reason to head to the slopes when we get them here.

I enjoy downhill skiing, but like cross country skiing on a golf course, I find wide open slopes with perfectly groomed terrain boring. I have no interest in corduroy. So I tend to downhill ski on a day when there's enough snow to make it interesting. Then I look for things on the trail that make the downhill trip more fun. I have never understood the skiers who try to get in as many runs as possible, zipping down the hill as fast as they can just to spend another 10 or 15 or 20 minutes on the lift. Again it's the American problem of valuing quantity over quality. I don't want a maximum number of runs per day, I want the maximum amount of fun per lift ride.

I learned about looking for fun on the trail by accident one day as I skied behind a boy of about 8 or 10 years old. As he went down, he scoured the mountain for every little change in terrain or pile of snow that could give him a nice little dip or even some "air." As I skied right behind him, I realized he was getting a lot more fun out of the trail than everyone else racing to the lift line. Have you ever noticed those little paths through the trees off to the side of the trail? They're made by kids having fun. You have to slow down to enjoy them, but as the saying goes, "the day is long and the pay is low" so what's your hurry?

As you might expect, I don't ski with a helmet. No one my age grew up skiing with a helmet and even when I was a young adult helmets were not common on the slopes. Then again, I'm not doing anything that extreme. If I ski narrow ungroomed trails or through the trees, which I do because it's more fun and interesting than skiing wide-open perfectly groomed trails, I choose less steep terrain and go slowly, especially the first time though, a much safer plan than putting on a helmet and skiing like a madman. It seems to me that if you have to put on so much clothing and gear to protect you from the elements that you are essentially inside, you lose the benefit of being outdoors.

It is ironic that as equipment has improved and trails have been widened and groomed to perfection, it takes bigger and steeper mountains for skiing to remain challenging and interesting. A few years ago, John and I got snowboards after taking a lesson while on a downhill ski trip. We spent several weekend days in April trying them out on a very small ski hill less than an hour from Boston. We later took them to other small ski resorts nearby that we had long since outgrown on our skis. We were more than sufficiently challenged and far from bored. Trying a new sport in effect "gave us back" those little local hills. And so does a good dump of snow. We have found that if we can get to the mountain just after a good snowfall, even the small local hill is challenging and fun and a lot less crowded than a big resort.

Now we ski or snowboard depending on the conditions. Snowboards are particularly good in deep powder or during the spring when the snow gets heavy and wet. I do not recommend snowboards, particularly for a novice, when the snow is very hard packed or icy. If you do try a snowboard for the first time, wear a helmet. Yes you read that right! You will most certainly fall while you are learning, and unlike skiing, there is something about snowboarding that causes you to give your head a good hard whack whenever you do.

This past winter in late March one of my cousins visited from Ireland with his wife and two kids. None of them had ever skied before and we hoped to get a day at our local ski mountain when they could give it a try. As the visit approached, John kept an eye on the weather forecast and it looked like there would be one beautiful day in the week, sunny and 30°F, a perfect ski day. Unfortunately, my cousins had made hotel reservations in the city for the night before, and wouldn't make it to the mountain 'til the following day, which didn't look so good. We decided to stick to our plan and offered to take the kids with us while their parents remained in town. The day was unbelievable, warm and sunny with perfect snow, and after a lesson and some practice on the bunny slope, both of the kids made it up the chairlift and down the green trail, a substantial accomplishment for the first day out. As forecasted, the following day was cold and rainy. I very much doubt if the trip would have been as successful if we had waited. Both of the kids had a blast and can't wait to go skiing again. We got the day for Dingle and we took it.

This year when we took our annual spring trip to Ireland, we had a lovely bike ride around Dingle peninsula on an unusually sunny, warm day. As John says, "For some reason it's always sunny in Dingle and it always rains when you're shopping in Killarney."

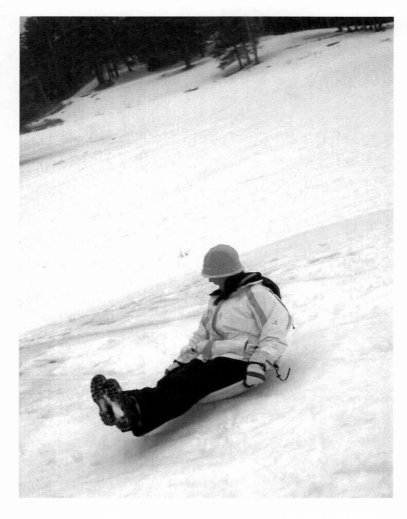

Sledding

4. Sledding

Chances are, unless you have small children, you haven't been sledding in years. I will say up front that children seem to be a necessary accessory for sledding. But that doesn't have to be the case, and even if it were, you could probably rustle up one or two who would be delighted to go with you. We don't have children, but we have plastic sleds of various sizes in our garage (mostly picked up at tag sales and swap shops), and since we get a lot of snow, quite a few visiting nieces and cousins have had their first, but not their last, sledding experiences with us.

I have no idea why sledding has become just a children's activity. Old novels (like Edith Wharton's, *Ethan Frome*) suggest that before easy access to movies and ski lifts, sledding was also enjoyed at least by young and single adults. That was certainly the case when I was in college, though it required some improvisation. When it snowed we went "traying," as opposed to sledding, down the Divinity School hill. (I never saw any Divinity School students out there, just us undergraduates, so maybe even then there was some age limit or maybe it was the serious nature of their studies.) The trays we used were the heavy plastic dining hall trays that we all used to collect our cafeteria style meals. When it snowed, we conveniently forgot to return them on our way out the door. After dinner we would head up the hill and "tray" down. It was a great hill except for the fact that it ended rather abruptly at a wrought iron fence next to the street, resulting in more than a few rough landings when it was icy, which it was much of the time.

Through it all the dining hall staff were philosophical. After the first day of snow when they realized that the trays were going missing, they put up a sign:

Do not remove trays.

After another day or two they put up a new sign:

Please return
dining hall trays.

On the third day, having not gotten much response to the first two signs, they put a pile of chipped trays by the entrance under a third sign:

Please use chipped
trays for traying!

One has to admire their pragmatism and it does make the point that while you do need something on which to slide down the hill, it needn't be fancy.

If you live where there's snow, sledding is about as low cost, low key, and low carbon as you can get while still having an exhilarating time. In New England there's always some local hill where people gather when conditions are right, often the first tee of the nearest golf course. It doesn't have to be that big a hill, particularly as the snow gets packed down and becomes faster and given that for every ride down, there is the strenuous and warming hike up, dragging your sled, toboggan and/or three-year-old behind you. Climbing stairs may be good exercise, but let's face it, after climbing the stairs up to your office all you get to do is work – not much of a pay off compared with sliding down the hill!

Of course, like all other natural outdoor activities, sledding is real, not an amusement park ride that someone else has designed for you, so you need to decide for yourself when, where and how it's safe to play. As simple as it looks, sledding can be dangerous. (If you don't think so, go back and read *Ethan Frome*!) I have no doubt that some adults, particularly women, consciously or unconsciously avoid sledding and other childhood games, like jumping off diving boards, because they're afraid. But of course if it weren't a little scary it wouldn't be as fun and exciting, and if you haven't done something like that in a while, it can be pretty exhilarating. That said, sledding doesn't have to be dangerous if you pay attention to the conditions and adjust your behavior accordingly. That doesn't mean sitting inside the house waiting for "perfect" conditions. It does mean paying attention to whether the snow is thick and slow or perhaps, after a few days, becoming icy and slick. There's little chance of hurting oneself when the snow is deep and fluffy, but as it gets packed down or even icy, you'll want to avoid hitting a bump the wrong way and tumbling off the toboggan.

If you do bring children sledding, it's obviously the responsibility of the adults to make sure they are doing it safely. If conditions are slick, walk the child halfway down the hill before getting on the sled to go to the bottom. As you become more comfortable with the conditions you'll know exactly how high up you can start to have a fun, safe run.

My three-year-old niece is not terribly stoic when confronted with challenging or adverse conditions so we weren't too sure how she'd take to sledding. For one thing she doesn't like the cold and is quick to tell us she wants to go inside because it's "too chilly." So for her first day out we picked a nice sunny warmish (for winter) day and made sure she was all dressed up in snowsuit, mittens and hat. Then we carefully scoped out the hill looking for a nice gentle slope for her first trip down. Because it was slick, I walked her halfway down the hill before letting her go down to the bottom where my brother was waiting to catch her. One time I walked too far down and by the time I let go, the sled didn't go very far before stalling. "Chilly" was not impressed. She turned around to look at me and said, "Faster!" A successful first outing – leave 'em begging for more!

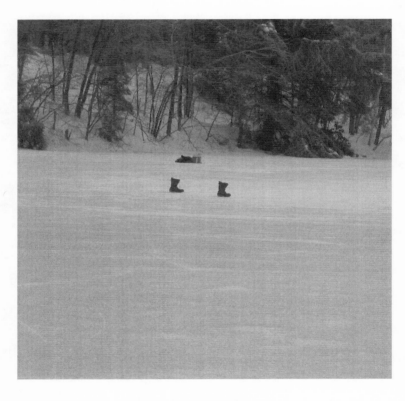

Impromptu goal posts

5. Ice Skating

Most winters we have a least a few weeks of cold dry weather that's perfect for ice skating. Even more than sledding, you have to get it while you can because at any moment you can have a thaw or a major snowstorm that puts an end to the skating.

These days most people have never ice skated on natural ice. The hockey players have a special name for their sport played on natural ice – "pond hockey." There's actually a pond hockey tournament in New Hampshire every winter. I've even seen articles that refer to skating on natural ice as "wild" ice skating. That seems a little dramatic. I never thought of ice skating as an extreme sport.

Then again the drama may be warranted. People are so unused to skating on natural ice that they don't know how to assess the conditions and are, therefore, always afraid. One day a couple of winters ago, I took my two nieces ice skating on what was really a large puddle in a town park. It was a Saturday and there was one other family there, a dad and two small kids learning to skate with plastic crates. It was a beautiful sunny day in January and it had been very cold for two weeks so there was plenty of ice everywhere, including on this little puddle. No sooner had we gotten there than a police cruiser pulled up. Someone in one of the houses across the street had called to report this suspicious activity! I have never been much of a demonstrator, but I was prepared to risk arrest that day to defend our right to ice skate outdoors. Fortunately, my brother, who is a member of the town fire department and teaches ice rescue courses in the Connecticut River, was able to assure the officer that conditions were fine.

Whoever called the police that day did so out of ignorance. Ignorance is typically a pejorative term used to describe country people who lack formal education. But the term applies equally to educated people who lack practical knowledge that in previous generations was gained from elders and experience. Most of us, including me, know very little about nature out our own back doors. Indeed, through mass media and television we are more likely to know about tsunamis in the South Pacific than about ordinary natural phenomena at home.

I grew up skating outdoors on local ponds where the ice skating was supervised by the town recreation department. I knew how to assess the conditions. You called a special telephone number and listened to the recording to see if the pond was open for skating! My mother, being from Ireland, was not a swimmer and was unfamiliar with ice and so was afraid of anything to do with the water. As a result, she diligently took us to swimming lessons and insisted on supervised ice skating. There was a small pond right down the street from our house, but since it wasn't supervised by the town, we couldn't skate there (unless my father, who grew up in New England, took us when he got home). Naturally, being somewhat forbidden, it was very exciting.

The sad thing is that like all ignorance, ignorance of the natural world makes us afraid and fear limits what we can do. It's ironic that at the same time that modern technology, such as air travel, apparently expands our opportunities abroad, ignorance of the natural world where we live contracts our opportunities at home. No doubt some people will say it's worth the trade-off, but I disagree. Whether it's a trip to a ski resort or a package deal to Cancun, you might as well buy a ticket for an amusement park ride where everything is thought out for you and all you have to do is show up. Step outside that package deal, however, and you will find a world of challenge and adventure in your own backyard or, in this case, on your local pond.

So how do you know if the ice is safe? There's nothing wrong with a recorded message if your town offers supervised ice skating and if it doesn't, and you get the weather for it, you might consider suggesting that it should.

Like the walk to school movement that has started to take
off in some places, old fashioned ideas are gaining purchase
these days. Barring that, marry a Boy Scout. I did and it's
come in handy more than once. The Boy Scout rule is still
good law:

> 1 inch no way
>
> 2 inches one may play
>
> 3 inches two may play
>
> 4 inches all may play

It also pays to be familiar with your own area.
Observe the ponds near you during the winter, which are
first to freeze, where there are inlets and outlets which may
stay open all year. Since we live on a spring fed lake, we
need to be aware of the locations of the springs, as the ice
over them may never freeze as solidly as that on the rest of
the lake.

You also need to pay attention to the weather. In
New England, there are always ice skating accidents in
December. Here, December is rarely cold enough for ice
skating. But as January and February go by we invariably
have several days at a time when the temperature doesn't get
above freezing. Just then, when everyone else is making

reservations for Acapulco, you can safely be digging out your ice skates. Finally, and this is the easiest test of all, notice where the ice has been shoveled clear and the kids are playing hockey. If the ice is holding up six to eight kids a side, you can be pretty sure it's safe for one or two more.

There are advantages to skating on natural ponds that you might not expect. For one thing it's easier to skate on natural ice than on glassy rink ice made even slipperier by the sheet of water laid down by the Zamboni. Natural ice often has some snow on top or mixed in with it that gives you something to grip with your skates. My five-year-old niece who had been taking skating lessons on an indoor rink found it much easier to stay upright when we went out on the lake.

Of course it practically goes without saying that skating outdoors on a pond simply does not compare to skating on rink ice in a man-made setting, particularly if it's indoors (although you can have a lot of fun on an outside man-made rink if you have access to one). Our lake is a deep spring fed lake that is the last to freeze in our area. When it does freeze, it's often buried in snow so deep that ice skating really isn't possible, so we have to make the most of it when conditions are right. Last winter we had just such a week in February and John and I went out on our skates. We were the only two out there on a lake a mile long and half a mile wide and in the shadow of a nearby mountain. Although we swim in the lake and row on it all summer, somehow that makes it even more amazing to literally walk on water in January. But it was also a little scary. There were cracks in the ice through which we could see that the ice was probably more than a foot deep, but every now and then we would hear a huge gurgle beneath our feet as the ice "settled" and an underwater wave traversed the lake. I began to wonder if we were crazy.

Just then a neighbor pulled up in his truck and came walking out on the ice towards us. I half expected him to warn us off, but instead, he said he'd seen us out skating and came out to see if he should call a group of friends he played hockey with to tell them to come down here instead of meeting at a local rink. The next thing we knew hockey players began arriving, sitting out on the ice to put on their skates and setting out snow boots for goalposts. The game was on. Shortly after that another group of neighbors we hadn't seen in months appeared with their skates. It was as if Brigadoon appeared out of the mist for just that afternoon. A reporter for the community paper happened by and took a picture. A couple of days later a snowstorm blew in and the ice disappeared once again – until next time.

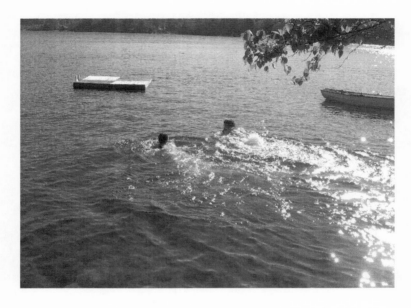

Swimming to the raft

Summer

1. Swimming

Bathing is an undescribed luxury. To feel the wind blow on your body, and the water flow upon you and lave you, is a rare physical enjoyment this hot day.

> — H.D. Thoreau, Journals *Summer*, July 9, 1852

People from Ireland generally are not good in heat. In Ireland anything above 75°F is considered a "scorcher." My mother minded the heat terribly when she first came to the United States and she didn't exactly come to the hottest part of it. I seem to have inherited those genes. On a trip to Indonesia some years ago, I was really only comfortable at the top of an old volcano where it was misty and 50°F.

So when it got hot in the summer my mother took us swimming – swimming lessons in the morning, recreational swimming in the afternoon. We swam at local town pools and ponds where Red Cross swimming lessons were given.

We also took day trips and vacations to the beach. Today, I spend summers on a lake in New Hampshire and my hair is wet from June to September (and that's not by accident).

The hottest days of summer, like the coldest days of winter, require a change in schedule to enjoy outdoor exercise. During the coldest and shortest days of winter, I find myself sleeping later in the morning and generally try to get outside and exercise in the middle of the day when the sun is brightest. When the days really start to lengthen in spring, I find myself bouncing out of bed bright and early, and by the time summer comes, I am outside swimming or bike riding mornings and evenings and spend the hottest part of the day working indoors or in the shade.

Most cities and towns have natural or man-made lakes and ponds or swimming pools that are open to the public in the summer. Even in the middle of downtown Boston, I can ride my bike across town after work and swim at a beautiful South Boston Beach where, thanks to the Harbor Clean Up project, the water is as clean as that at the suburban beaches many miles north or south of the city.

Unlike most other sports and outdoor activities, swimming involves getting used to an entirely different environment, which may take some time. Every year when I start swimming again in early summer it takes a little while to get used to having my face in the water and not being able to breathe all the time. It takes time to get back into the rhythm of stroking and breathing, quite apart from getting used to the physical activity itself.

I confess that as a former life guard and swimming instructor, I am biased towards swimming and think it is a great activity that everyone should learn to do properly. Not only does swimming keep you cool in the summer, it's a great form of exercise. It doesn't stress leg joints, like knees and ankles, and so is a great alternative to running, tennis and hiking, particularly if you have an injury.

Even when I was growing up and there were plenty of mothers at home to take kids to local swimming lessons, many kids stopped taking lessons after a session or two and never learned to swim well enough to use swimming as a regular form of exercise as adults. These days, with fewer parents at home even during the summer, the situation is probably worse. All I can say is, if your child attends a summer camp, make sure it's one that teaches kids to swim well enough that they will be able do it for exercise, as well as for fun, all their adult lives.

If you know how to swim but have never swum for exercise, next summer get out there and give it a try. Start in the summer, outdoors, when it's hot, and late enough in the year that the water has had a chance to warm up. At the risk of stating the obvious, swimming is a lot more attractive on a hot day. Warm up before you go in by running, playing tennis, doing yard work or anything that makes you so hot you want to go for a swim. Hint, even if it's not blazing hot, you'll get warm enough from running a mile or two to want to jump in. When we went to the beach in Maine as kids, my father always had us run up and down the beach (preferably barefoot with our feet in the water to get used to it) before diving in, a particularly good idea in Maine where even in August the water temperature may not get out of the 50s.

While I love the ocean, I never actually swim in the waves. I do my swimming in the calmer waters of pools, ponds or lakes. If you're swimming in a chlorinated pool, I definitively recommend goggles to avoid the chlorine's irritating or drying out your eyes. Once you start and after you've had a chance to get used to the environment you should naturally be able to increase your distance with experience. If you're swimming in a lake or pond or at the beach, and have a destination, such as a raft or buoy, even better.

For all my lessons and experience, I wouldn't say that I am a terribly strong swimmer. My strokes look good, but just aren't that effective. My sister, on the other hand, seems to cover more distance with one stroke than I do in ten. I did pick up a tip last year that seems to have helped (one is never too old to learn) and that is to kick. I don't think I ever really bothered kicking before and my sister is a diligent kicker so I thought it was worth a try and it is!

If you never learned how to swim or simply can't remember proper strokes, take lessons. This is a tall order. It's not easy to learn to swim as an adult and swimming lessons, whether indoor or out, invariably occur in less than enticing weather. But if you want to invest your time and effort in something that will make your life more enjoyable and healthier, consider swimming lessons. Remember, it will take time to get comfortable with it, so don't quit just because you're not having fun after one or two sessions. Also make sure to get yourself outdoors swimming on a hot day, preferably at a lake or pond or at the beach, so you can see the payoff. After you do successfully learn to swim the length of the dock or pool, go ahead and jump in!

Once a year, a local group meets at 8 am on a Saturday morning to swim across the lake, a distance of about a mile. The lake swim occurs in mid August after both the lake and the swimmers have had a chance to warm up. About 30 or 40 people show up each year, ranging in age from 8 to 80. There's also a flotilla of boats following along in case anyone runs into trouble. My sister usually does the swim with me and John and my nieces follow in the rowboat. My nieces are both taking swimming lessons and looking forward to the day they can do the swim too. The highlight is the blueberry pancake breakfast after the swim. See you there.

2. Tennis

I like tennis and have played more or less every summer since I was a kid, mostly just batting the ball back and forth with friends on local public courts, and trying with more or less success to keep out of the way of the serious tennis ladies in their official outfits. I've taken some lessons as an adult, but I've never gotten into an organized league. There was no question that I would include tennis as a summer (or spring or fall) outdoor activity, but I sensed a certain lack of enthusiasm (on my part) as I readied to put pen to paper. So like any good lawyer about to make an argument, I tried to identify the problem and address it head on.

The problem with tennis, I decided, is that you have to have someone with whom to play. It's not like swimming that you can either do on your own or with other people. And the real problem is, you can't play tennis with just anyone. Tennis isn't golf where, even though you may play in a foursome, everyone is playing their own game. In order for tennis to "work" the players on opposite sides of the net have to be of reasonably similar abilities. Yes, comparable abilities are helpful if people are biking, running or hiking together, though John and I have developed a few tricks to get around differing abilities in those areas, but biking and running you can always do on your own and one person's experience is not totally dependent on another person's performance.

In tennis, on the other hand, if one player hits 90 mile an hour line drives and the other gently lobs the ball, neither can play with the other. It's not a question of right or wrong, or nice or mean. It's simply the fact that your shot comprises 50% what you put into it and 50% what it had on it coming over the net. (I once hit one of the best winners of my life by simply sticking out my racket and letting a young kid's line drive ricochet back at him.) And of course no one is having fun if the ball can't be kept in play.

This is probably why people, and particularly ladies, are either into tennis and play regularly at a club or with a regular group or don't play at all. For the former, this seems to result in a sort of tennis arms race where everyone takes more and more lessons, gets bigger and better rackets and plays more and more tennis to keep up with the group (at least until they get injured). The inevitable result is playing tennis year round, indoors in the wintertime here in the Northeast, an obvious conflict with my philosophy of enjoying a variety of activities seasonally, outdoors.

But before we give up on tennis altogether, let's consider some of its advantages. First and foremost, it's accessible. Before the widespread building of public tennis courts in the 1970s, tennis was largely a rich person's game. The only tennis courts were at private country clubs or a very few houses. All of that changed when I was a kid. Public tennis courts were built pretty much everywhere and tennis was available to anyone who could get her hands on an inexpensive racket.

We take that for granted now, but compare sports which are still largely only available to people with lots of money. Horseback riding springs immediately to my mind, since I love riding my half a horse and might even ride a whole one if the cost weren't prohibitive. As great an outdoor activity as it is, riding is simply too expensive for the average family with a couple of kids who don't want to devote all of their resources to a horse. Downhill skiing has become more accessible over the years, but is still a very expensive sport even if you live within driving distance of the mountain. Sailing is another activity that apart from a few public programs, is largely restricted to private clubs and members who can afford to join them. So now those free tennis courts in the local park are looking pretty good, and as you're probably paying for them with your taxes, you're thinking you should get out there and use them.

Another plus, tennis lends itself to flattering attire (compare ice hockey or roller blading). I don't generally wear official tennis clothes, and you will be fine in shorts and a T-shirt. I buy "cheerleader skirts" popular with teens at regular stores and get lots of compliments from the serious tennis ladies wearing tennis shop attire. (You can buy shorts or trunks to go under the skirt with a pocket to hold an extra ball.) I have never liked the look of visors, so if it's sunny, I wear a straw hat playing tennis (the same one I wear bike riding or sailing) and yes it generates a lot of comments (mostly nice). It's a better look for me and tells the world (and more importantly anyone who might be thinking of playing with me) that I have no Olympic aspirations, I'm there just to have fun. If you do happen to hit a winner, you may catch your opponent by surprise – at least the first time!

So now you're ready to go out and play. As with everything pick a nice day. If you've read this far, you know that every day is a nice day for something, so pick a nice day for tennis, ideally one of the first warm days of spring when you can actually go outside without long underwear. If you haven't been playing regularly, find someone who's in the same boat and head out to the courts. Don't limit yourself to regulation games, especially at the beginning. I myself have spent years "rallying," simply hitting the ball back and forth from the baseline and not bothering with serving or keeping score. As I may have said before, I enjoy running after the ball at least as much as I enjoy hitting it and you get more exercise from 45 minutes of singles rallying than from most doubles matches.

If you have an opportunity to take some lessons or a local clinic, take it. As with any sport or game, a few lessons at the beginning can help get you more quickly to the stage where you're having fun. But be forewarned: particularly with tennis I've noticed that lessons come in two flavors, the really hard but right way to do it if you're going to the Olympics and the short cut way to quickly become effective and keep the ball in play. You want the short cuts, every short cut you can get! After years of struggling to serve (and hence get though a game) using the traditional wind up that ideally requires a 6' 2" frame (which John has, but sadly I lack by nearly a foot), a young woman instructor who'd starred on her college tennis team and, more importantly, was no taller than I, showed me a much more straightforward serve that has served me well (no pun intended) ever since. You can also learn some basic strategies that increase the odds of keeping the ball in play, literally which shots are long shots and which are a more of sure thing.

Lessons or clinics are also a good way to meet people who may just be getting started or back into the sport and are looking for people with whom to play. I have also found that some of the drills used at clinics can be fun to play on your own instead of or in addition to regular games.

Notwithstanding everything I said above, there are ways to have fun and get some exercise even if you are playing with people of different abilities. That's actually where drills come in handy. Drills usually require one person to place the ball in a certain quadrant of the opposite court to allow the other player to try to execute a certain shot, for example, an approach shot and then a volley at the net. Even though the volleyer is the person being "drilled," it's actually pretty challenging to be the person on the other side of the net trying to place the ball accurately where the volleyer is supposed to hit it. A good instructor makes that part look easy, but it's not!

For the recreational player, accuracy and control can be as important and effective as the hard-hitting that is the holy grail of regular club and indoor players. Think of the older ladies and gentlemen who appear to hit the ball softly but, by putting it exactly where they want it, win more games than you might expect. Even those who like to hit the ball hard and have a nice big racket that helps them do so, can take a day to work on finesse and placement if they are playing with a kid or someone who doesn't hit the ball as hard as they do.

Even if you are not that serious a player and have spent a good portion of your hour on the court doing drills or rallying, you should work up to playing a few games. Actual games will allow you to practice your serve, practice your return of serve, and focus on keeping the ball inside the lines, a requirement that can easily go by the wayside when you're just rallying. Just because it's a game, however, doesn't mean you can't rig it a little bit to keep the ball in play and have more fun.

Ladies tennis has a great thing called "FBI" which means that the player returning serve will return the server's "first ball in" and prior missed serves will not be counted. Again, no one has fun if the server is losing every point by double faulting. We are out there to get some exercise as well as have some fun and winning will not achieve that objective if no one gets a racket on the ball (or a ball to run after)! Even if you are inexperienced, you may have more success in a game than you might think. Over the years I have won many games against John by simply keeping the ball in the court, his otherwise hard-hit winners failing to stay inside the lines - that, plus a certain diplomacy on his part that most husbands would be wise to emulate. (As he says, "I wasn't married yesterday.")

Unless you live in Florida, tennis is not a winter sport. It can be fun to stretch the season by wearing leggings under your short skirt and a sweater over your top, but once the leaves start to fall, hang up your racket until next year. After all, you wouldn't want to miss the first cross country ski day for a pre-scheduled tennis match inside a bubble. Nor do you want to miss the first day of tennis next spring because you never had a last day of tennis last fall.

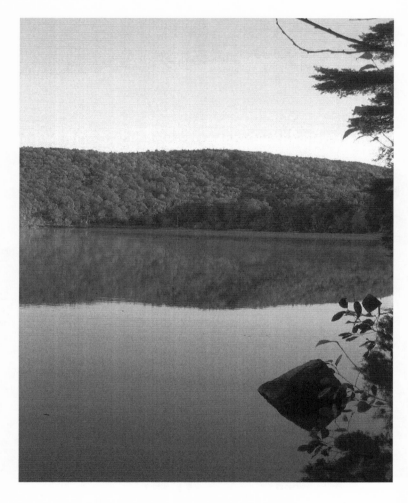

New Hampshire lake on a still day

3. On the Water – Rowing, paddling, sailing

Particularly because I mind the heat, I like to spend as much of the summer as possible in, on or near the water. If you live somewhere that's really hot, the water may be the only real option for outdoor activity in the summer. There is nothing like being on the water to give a fresh perspective to things on shore, even if they are only a few feet away. Of course to have fun on the water you need to be able to handle yourself in the water, so learn to swim (see above).

Getting out on the water can be as simple or as complicated as you like. Most of us have taken a canoe out on a pond or quiet river with parents, at camp or on a school outing. Canoes are often available for the price of admission at ponds and lake beaches. Our local Audubon Society has canoes that any member can take out to go birding or just to paddle up and down the river. Almost every substantial river (and many not so substantial ones) has an outfit that will not only rent you a canoe for the day, but will drop you off up river and pick you up downstream so you get an extended ride – what John who grew up in Missouri calls a "float trip."

From the look of things, it seems as though kayaks have surpassed canoes as the easiest, low-cost way to get out on the water and no doubt they have some substantial advantages. They are light, very portable and can be operated easily by one person. They are also relatively inexpensive to buy or rent and not difficult to learn how to use if you plan to stay in calm waters. I've tried kayaking, and it was okay, but I prefer a canoe. I don't like sitting that low in the water and I especially don't like having my lower body trapped inside the plastic shell (indeed, the whole thing is a little too plastic for me). In a canoe you sit up higher (I know the Indians knelt, but I'm not an Indian). Also I like the fact that John and I can go out together in one canoe (we would need two kayaks) and we can even throw a third person (like a child) in the middle. But whichever you prefer, canoeing and kayaking are readily accessible and if you've never been out on the water and would like to get started, either of them is a good choice.

John and I took a number of canoe trips with the outing club in college. A group of us headed south for spring break and spent a week on a river or in the Everglades camping out every night. More recently, we have done week long trips with a group of neighbors down the wilderness waterway in Allagash State Park in Maine. Although I didn't realize it at the time, canoe camping trips appealed to me, where backpacking trips did not, because with the canoe, I didn't have to carry all the stuff on my back. The trips were a blast. Even though I had no canoeing experience at all prior to my first trip, others in the group did and were able to teach me the basic strokes. Also, the river trips were downstream where the river itself provided a good part of the momentum. One did have to learn to steer the current, which made the whole thing much more interesting, and it's really not that difficult to do if you choose a fairly gentle stream. (If your basic 10 year old kid at camp can learn to do it, how difficult can it be?)

Still, both in Florida and in Maine, there were several large lakes that had to be crossed, inevitably upwind, which tested the limits of my modest upper body strength. Necessity being the mother of invention, John and I figured out that if we ever wanted to get where we were going, we needed to put him in the bow (otherwise known as "the engine room"). So while John paddled hard, switching sides every few strokes, I would angle my paddle every now and then to keep us on an even keel.

Whenever I see a couple, a man and a woman, out in a canoe on a Saturday or Sunday afternoon, inevitably the guy is in the stern. Presumably he knows more about canoeing, having done it as a Boy Scout, and thinks he's the only one who can steer. But the truth is steering is not that hard and is physically a lot less demanding than just plain paddling. So assuming the man is the physically stronger of the two, it makes no sense to have him in the stern and her in the bow. Why should he get to take a break every couple of strokes to steer while she has to keep paddling? (Yes, I know one can paddle and steer at the same time, but you will get a lot more out of the guy if he is up front just paddling than if he is in the back trying to steer too.) While John and I initially took some ribbing for our seat positions, the truth is we could never have kept up with the group if he had spent half of his time steering instead of paddling.

I also love to sail, having sailed dinghies in college and larger boats as an adult. Unless you're hiking out in a dinghy, I'm not sure there's much exercise involved, but sailing does give you a great feeling of being outdoors. Also, since you have to be aware of the speed and direction of the wind, and in some locations the current and tide, it gives you an awareness of nature that you would not otherwise have if getting where you were going didn't depend on it. Learning to sail is a little more complicated than paddling a canoe on a quiet pond, but it's a great thing to do if you have the opportunity at a camp or resort.

I should make clear that I am not talking about paying someone else to take you out for a paddle, row or sail. I am not talking about rafting trips down Class 5 rapids through the Grand Canyon where someone else is doing the driving. Neither a bus tour nor an amusement park ride bears any resemblance to learning to do something yourself and doing it. John and I once did Class 1 rapids in a canoe in Maine and I assure you Class 1 rapids on your own are way more exciting than Class 5 rapids when someone else is doing the driving.

For several years John and I were members of a sailing club in Boston and especially on hot nights we would pick up something for dinner after leaving the office and head down to the harbor to take out a boat. Once we got out of the inner harbor (after dodging the inevitable departing cruise ship as a 747 roared overhead coming in for a landing at Logan Airport), we would sail around the harbor islands leaving work and worry behind. Heading for home after the sun had set, we would watch the lights coming on in the office towers. Viewed from the water through the Rowes Wharf Archway, Boston never looked more beautiful.

Now, we are more likely to be out in a rowboat on the lake as the sun sets in the west and the moon rises in the east. In some respects the experiences couldn't be more different. But in the essentials, they are the same.

4. Team Sports - Soccer to Street Hockey

Unfortunately, I was born just a few years too early for organized girl's soccer in my town. There were no organized team sports for girls when I was a kid. I remember the first girl to play on a boy's Little League team, but she was the exception (and a very good athlete) not the rule. So, unlike my sister, 11 years younger than I, who started in the town league when she was six and played through high school, I have no soccer skills. Nevertheless, that has not stopped me from kicking the ball around from time to time.

Pickup soccer games were a popular evening pastime and social event when I was a young teenager visiting Ireland. There the "field" was actually a "field" (hopefully, one from which the cows had been absent for a while). Later, after I'd started working, a neighbor got me into a women's over 30 soccer league which was a lot of fun. Most of the players had more skills than I had, but I was willing to run after anything so that's what I did – and then immediately kicked the ball to someone else.

I would guess that there are many more organized team sports for adult men than for adult women, but that is changing. I know a woman in her 40s who is involved in a very popular ice hockey league for women in her town. Most of the women involved did not play hockey as kids, and while it's not a look to which I aspire, I admire them for getting out there and they are having a blast. I'm sure that with all the girls who have now grown up playing soccer, there are more adult women's soccer leagues as well. I know there are women's softball leagues but I have always wondered, not being a softball player myself, whether there was any exercise involved. Obviously, you're most likely to be comfortable playing a team sport if you've played it as a kid and learned the basic skills. On the other hand, if you're relatively fit and the league is not too serious, you can probably join in and have a good time without too much trouble.

The one problem with team sports is that you have to have a team, actually two teams, to play the game, unless you modify the rules as in "seven aside" soccer, where they make do with one team by splitting it into two. If, like me, you are not an organizer, you have to hope someone in your area has organized a regular game. If you are an organizer, then do the rest of us a favor and organize! A group of neighbors has a regular Sunday morning (no traffic) street hockey game that meets all winter, weather permitting. It's organized by a guy who always seems to do the organizing and I'm sure the other players are grateful. With email, putting these things together has gotten a lot easier than when you had to telephone everyone individually, as long as you don't spend all your time twittering about it, but actually pick a place and time and get out there and do it!

Like raking leaves or shoveling snow, team sports are best enjoyed in season. Even if it's only once a week, that's a substantial commitment and you will be glad to hang up your cleats or skates at the end of the season and enjoy a change in routine.

Even if you never join or organize a local league, think about suggesting a pick up soccer game at your next family reunion or holiday gathering. Soccer is probably the easiest game for everyone to join in, but touch football (á là the Kennedys) also comes to mind. It's a great way to work up an appetite for a special meal and it beats watching TV. This past fall, while my oldest niece was playing in a kids' soccer league, we played pick up soccer with the younger ones, four and two, who were hanging around watching. In no time at all we were throwing off jackets and sweaters, while everyone else on the sidelines was shivering. The two-year-old, in particular, thought it was just great that everyone was running around with her – and she was right!

12.

What's on Your Playlist?

This is not meant to be a definitive list. I simply offer examples, those with which I am most familiar at that, of putting into practice the general theory of regular, seasonal outdoor activity. For some this list will be under inclusive. There are a lot of things I've left out – sports like horseback riding, wonderful but expensive, outdoor activities like hunting and fishing, which involve differing amounts of physical activity but epitomize seasonality and awareness of nature, unofficial "play" like Frisbee and catch, hotbox and riding waves at the beach which, like sledding down a hill, are, or at least used to be, largely the province of children. Then of course there's golf, which is more of a game than a sport, but which gets you outside (though in a largely artificial environment) and active (sort of), at least if you walk the course.

For some this list will be over inclusive. If it never snows where you live, then much of the winter chapter will not literally apply (though the all important discussion of clothing probably will). But each of the preceding chapters illustrates basic principles that apply anytime you head outside to play, whether you're doing one of the activities discussed in this book or something else that may be on your list that isn't on mine. Like cooking from a well stocked pantry, with these principles in mind you can put together a fun, invigorating, safe trip outside in any weather and at any time:

✔ *You want the day for Dingle*

> Swim when it's hot, ice skate when the pond freezes over, ride your bike on a dry day, go shopping when it rains

✔ *Life is not an amusement park ride*

> You decide when, where and how to play

✔ *Life is not a no-risk proposition*

> Exercise good judgment while you exercise outside

✔ *Artfully write the test*

> Choose the right route for the right conditions and you will have the right response

✔ *Don't be a pack horse*

> Carry little or nothing on your back or in your hands, which you can do because

✔ *It doesn't have to take all day*

> Much less all weekend, go out for an hour or two, but

✔ *You can't squeeze it in*

> To the parking lot or the stairway or while working or watching TV

✔ *It's a perfect day for something*

> Figure out what and then go outside and do it

✔ *You're "the man"*

> Work out(side)

✔ *Play together*

> It's easier than you think

✔ *There's no bad weather, only bad clothes*

Wear the right ones and enjoy every day

✔ *There's no place like home*

Go out and explore yours

✔ *Have I been outside today?*

It's a simple question, and there's only one right answer. Say YES! and you're on your way to looking good, feeling good, sleeping well and being happy.

EPILOGUE

Although this book is focused on recreational activities, I don't mean to exclude serious athletes or even men! My guess is that most serious athletes concentrate on one or two sports. Even people who are not competitive athletes but exercise regularly, for whatever reason, seem to do the same thing every day, day in and day out. I suggest that even they will benefit, mentally and physically, from going outside and doing something new.

I also want to be clear, in case there is any doubt, that I am talking about vigorous activity. I may not be cycling 50 miles, but I do ride 10 or 15 or 25. I don't run marathons, but I do run 3 or 4 miles several times a week. I am not riding or running as fast as someone who is training to compete, but I do go at what, for me, is a good clip, with the result that I am reasonably tired at the end. I am not saying that you don't have to exert yourself, but that you don't have to be able to exert yourself at a semi-professional level to get enormous physical and mental benefits from regular outdoor exercise. On the contrary, the curve is steepest at the bottom: I get a much greater benefit from running 9 miles a week compared to running 0, than I would get from increasing the 9 to 19. What I have learned from doing it all my life is that a little goes a long way, and a little of a lot of things goes even further and is a lot more fun.

During the course of working on this project, I've talked to lots of people about exercising outside. I've been struck by how few people have said, "You know, I think you're wrong. It's really just as good, or even better, to exercise indoors." On the contrary, I've noticed that once people are reminded about going outside, it gets a toe hold on their list of "Things to do Today" and may even climb up a rung or two. For most people, going outside is not a completely foreign idea, just one that has retreated into a distant past or been relegated to special events and holidays.

Just as when we were kids, we seem to need permission to "go outside and play" and doubt it will be granted unless all our homework is done. But as adults, all our work is never done. I know that I've drawn more than a few raised eyebrows over the years as I headed outside for a swim or run, leaving a house full of people and things to do behind me. But I knew, even if those around me didn't, that I'd be better able to handle the work to be done, not to mention better company, for my trip outside. Just because it's play, doesn't mean it's not important. On the contrary, play is every bit as important as work, going outside every bit as worthwhile as whatever it is we do inside. Ask yourself, "Have I been outside today?" Then give yourself permission to make it a priority. See you outside!

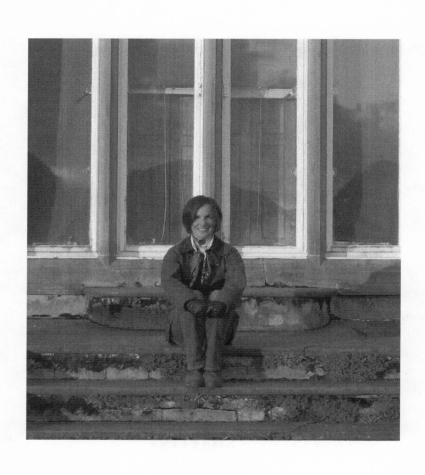

About the Author

Joan Griffin is a Boston trial attorney with over 20 years' experience trying civil and criminal cases. In her criminal practice, Joan earned national recognition for bringing the first successful challenge to the scientific basis of expert ballistics evidence. She is a popular speaker at forums nationwide on "Innovation vs. Inertia" based on her experience challenging forensic evidence. Joan has made frequent appearances on New England Cable News Network (NECN) providing analysis of high profile cases. She lives in New Hampshire and makes regular trips to Ireland visiting her extended family.